ASIAN BEAUTY

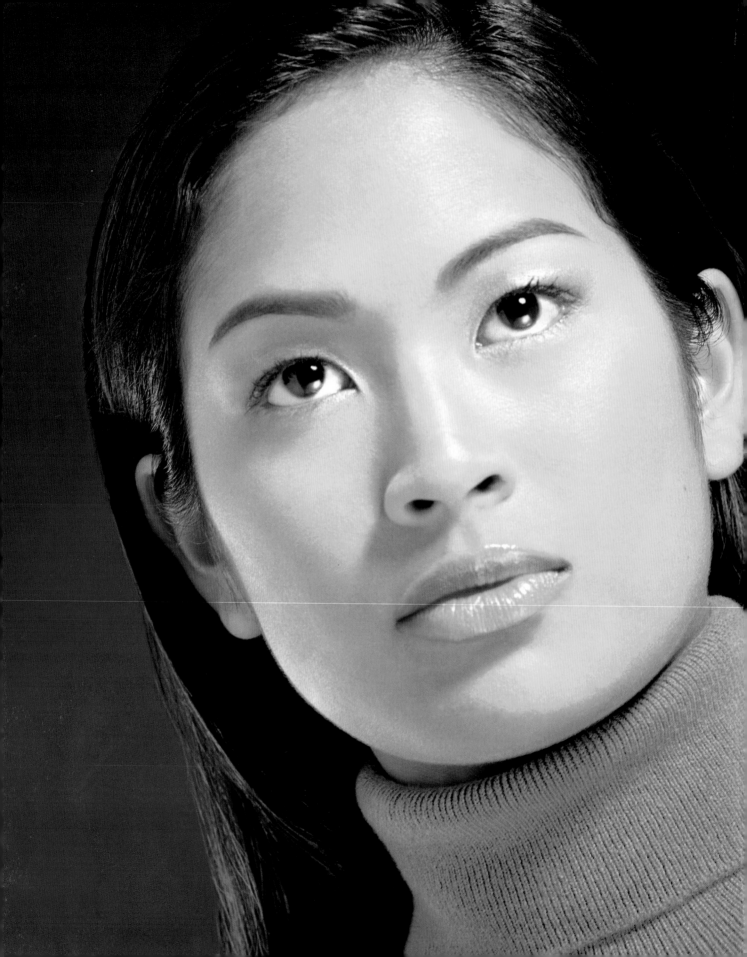

ASIAN BEAUTY

MARGARET KIMURA

with Marianne Dougherty

Photographs by Rich Marchewka

Still-Life photographs by Rich Marchewka and Toby Tilley

HarperResource
An Imprint of HarperCollins*Publishers*

HarperCollins books may be purchased for educational, business, or sales promotional use. For information, please write to: Special Markets Department, HarperCollins Publishers Inc., 10 East 53rd Street, New York, NY 10022.

FIRST EDITION

Still-life photographs copyright © 2001 Rich Marchewka Photography and Toby Tilley; all other photographs copyright © 2001 by Rich Marchewka Photography.

Book Design by Leah Carlson-Stanisic

Library of Congress Cataloging-In-Publication Data
Kimura, Margaret.
Asian beauty / Margaret Kimura with Marianne Dougherty.— 1st ed.
p. cm.
Includes index.
ISBN 0-06-018473-6
1. Beauty, Personal. 2. Women—Health and hygiene—Asia. I. Dougherty, Marianne. II. Title.

RA778 .K487 2001
646. 7'2'095—dc21

2001016669

01 02 03 04 05 TP 10 9 7 6 5 4 3 2 1

THIS BOOK IS DEDICATED TO MY FAMILY
AND IN LOVING MEMORY OF MY FATHER.

TO MY PARENTS WHO TRUSTED ME AT A VERY YOUNG
AGE TO GO OUT AND EXPLORE MY DREAMS.

TO MY TWO SISTERS AND MY BROTHER, YUMI, MARI, AND BILL,
WHO CONSTANTLY GAVE ME THE SUPPORT AND
ENCOURAGEMENT TO GO FOR IT.

AND TO LOLA, SAYDEE, AND OPIE,
WHO GAVE ME UNCONDITIONAL LOVE,
ESPECIALLY WHEN I REALLY NEEDED IT.

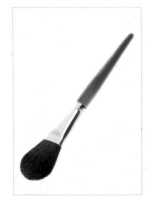
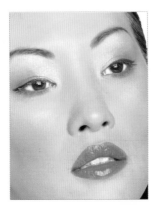
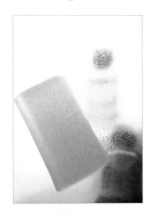

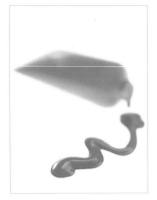
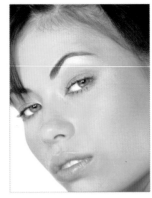
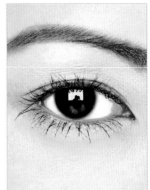

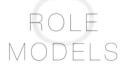
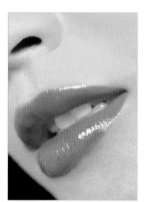
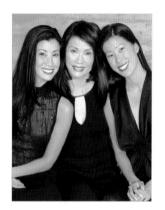
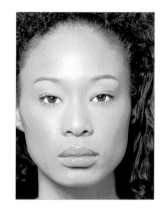
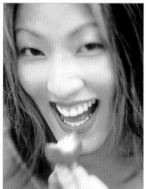
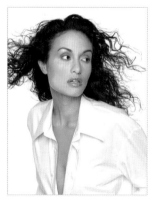
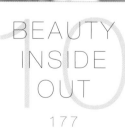

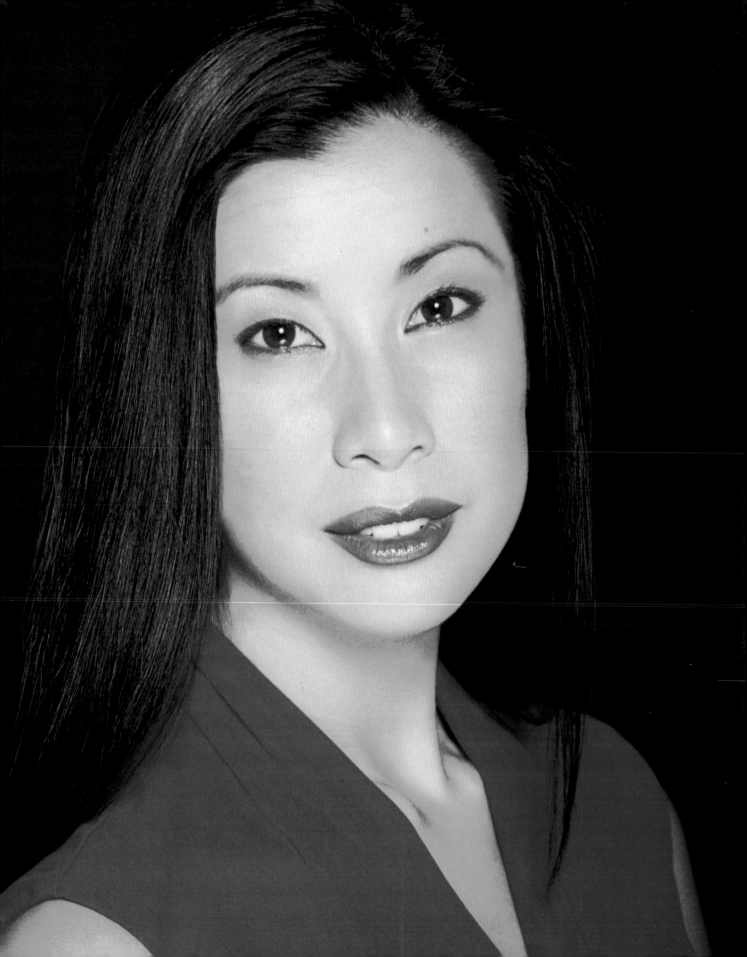

I'VE ALWAYS BEEN A POP CULTURE JUNKIE. LIKE SO MANY KIDS IN AMERICA, I WAS RAISED BY TELEVISION. THE FIRST THING I'D DO UPON RETURNING HOME FROM SCHOOL WAS SWITCH ON THE TV; THE IMAGES WOULD KEEP ME

ENTERTAINED UNTIL BEDTIME. EVEN AT A YOUNG AGE I WAS A VORACIOUS CONSUMER OF MAGAZINES: NEWS, FASHION, MUSIC, CELEBRITY, AND SO ON. DEEP DOWN I LONGED TO BE PART OF THE CULTURE INTO WHICH I WAS BORN, BUT SOMEHOW I NEVER FELT ENTIRELY COMFORTABLE. AS MUCH AS

I enjoyed watching *Three's Company* and *The Brady Bunch* or reading *Seventeen*, at a certain level I couldn't relate because I never saw anyone on those shows or in that magazine who looked anything like me. I remember wanting desperately to duplicate many of the looks featured in fashion magazines, scouring the beauty pages for makeup tips. Inevitably, my search would be in vain as none of the advice offered applied to people with my skin color and eyes like mine.

I learned everything I know about maintaining myself from the woman I consider the most beautiful in the world: my mother. She has always carried herself with elegance and confidence. Although I possess a minute fraction of the grace she exudes, at least I had someone from whom I could learn.

The climate in the media has changed since I was a child, but it still hasn't exactly been easy to find information about Asian beauty, until now. Margaret Kimura of Margaret Kimura Cosmetics has spent her career in the field of beauty. She had an ambitious dream of putting together a beautiful book that would give people an opportunity to learn more about and appreciate the great diversity that exists within the Asian community. Margaret's dream has finally become a reality as reflected in the following pages. This is a book that I wish I had had when I was a little girl, and one I will be proud to present to my own daughter one day.

— LISA LING

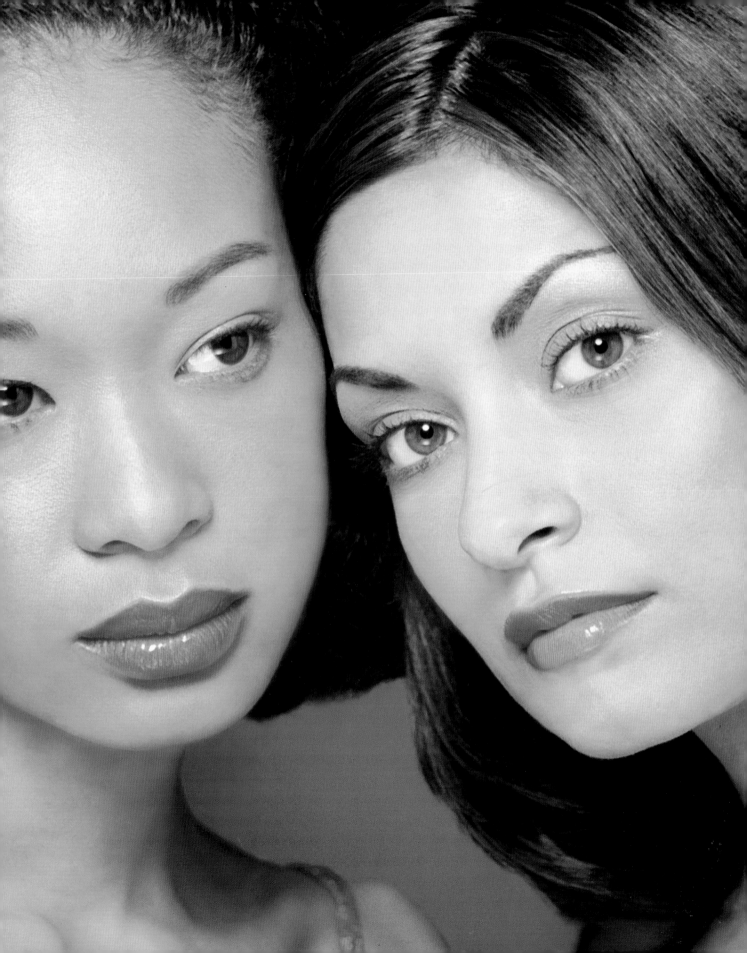

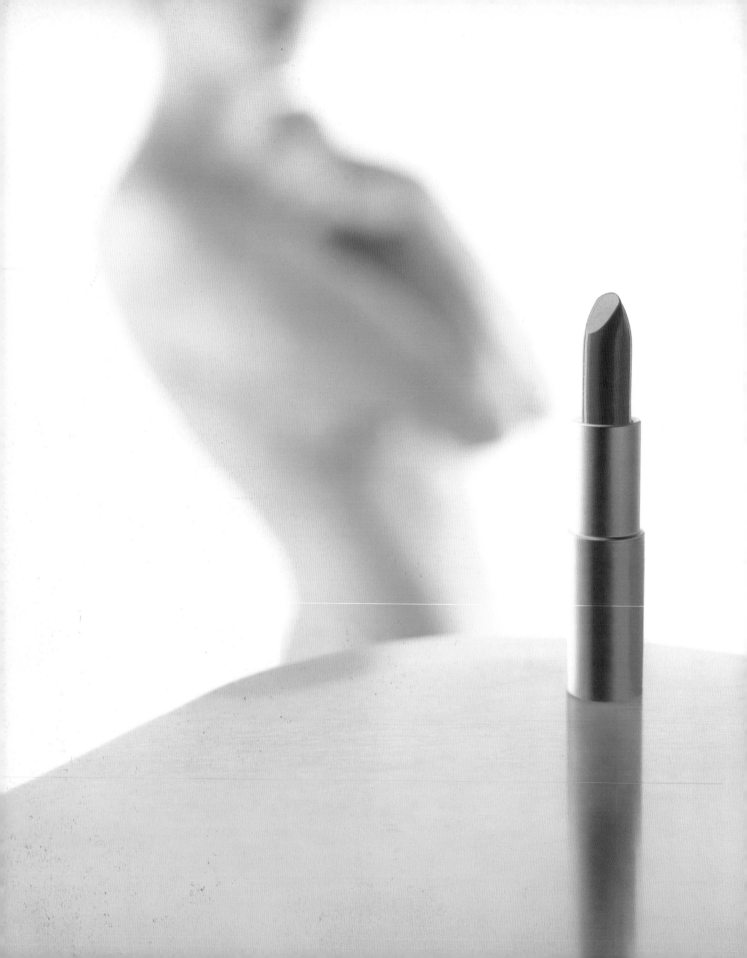

BEAUTY IS A SUBJECTIVE NOTION AT BEST, BUT THAT DOESN'T SEEM TO MATTER WHEN YOU'RE AN ASIAN-AMERICAN TEENAGER GROWING UP IN SOUTHERN CALIFORNIA, WHERE BEAUTY IS SYNONYMOUS WITH LONG BLONDE

INTRODUCTION

HAIR AND BLUE EYES. FINDING OUT WHERE I FIT INTO THE BEAUTY EQUATION TWENTY YEARS AGO WAS DIFFICULT AND PAINFUL AT BEST. THERE WEREN'T ANY ASIAN-AMERICAN MODELS IN THE PAGES OF *GLAMOUR* AND *SEVENTEEN*, AND NONE OF THE BEAUTY ADVICE I READ THERE SEEMED to apply to me. I suspect that for most beauty editors at that time Asian-American women were stereotyped as some kind of exotic cross between Suzie Wong and Madame Butterfly, which was almost the same as being invisible.

To further complicate matters, I had an athletic build, when everyone knows that "real Asian girls" have waiflike figures. At least that's what my mother always said. But I was an all-American girl who loved fast food as much as the next teenager, and I had the curves to prove it. I spent a lot of time and energy battling self-doubt and struggling to become comfortable with who I was, someone who fit neither the American nor the Asian beauty ideal. I had to invent my own idea of beauty, and my many years of experimentation led me to who I am today: a woman who is comfortable in her own body, and who appreciates the many diverse aspects of Asian-American beauty. The women featured in this book are a reflection of my idea of beauty: from Ann Lewis, who is Japanese and Irish, to Young, whose parents are Korean and African-American.

Nowadays there are a lot of Asian-American role models for young women to pattern themselves after, from Lisa Ling of *The View* to Lucy Liu, one of Charlie's twenty-first-century angels. Still, the pressure to conform to traditional standards of beauty can be enormous. Comedienne Margaret Cho got her own television show, then was warned by producers to slim down or else. Even more chilling, in Japan women actually have their eyelids surgically altered to look more Caucasian.

What I've come to realize is that cosmetics can play a significant role in how women perceive themselves, helping to shape our ideals of beauty and glamour. Makeup allows us to invent and reinvent ourselves, depending upon our mood, our age, our accomplishments, and even our sense of self-worth.

But there's something called inner beauty that's just as important. I learned that lesson from Audrey Hepburn, one of my early role models. When I was growing up, *Breakfast at Tiffany's* was one of my favorite movies, and I thought Audrey Hepburn was the most beautiful woman I'd ever seen. Then in the 1990s I had the privilege of working with her when she was doing a press junket for UNICEF. She was their spokesperson at the time, and I was impressed with how warm and caring she was. Absolutely nothing could prevent her from helping people in need.

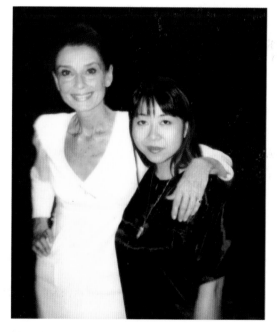

Here I am with my role model, Audrey Hepburn.

SHE WAS ALSO A GREAT LISTENER.

She looked right into your eyes when you spoke to her, AND SHE

SMILED AT YOU when you talked. *It just felt good to*

be in her presence. She made you feel like it was all right

to be yourself. There's no denying that she was a **BEAUTIFUL**

WOMAN, though she admitted that *she had never really thought*

of herself as a great beauty. Still, it was obvious that

HER BEAUTY WAS MORE THAN SKIN

DEEP. She exuded *courage, compassion,* and *incredible*

confidence. By the time I met her she was already in her sixties so

naturally she had lines on her face, but every one of them was

the kind you get around your eyes and mouth

from LAUGHING and SMILING too much.

I try to learn something new from everyone I meet. What I learned from Audrey was to look beneath the surface, for that's where real beauty resides. The English poet John Keats wrote, "Beauty is truth, truth beauty." As a makeup artist, it's my job to connect with the people in my chair, to see the truth of who they really are. Makeup merely gives them the confidence to speak that truth. That's beautiful to me.

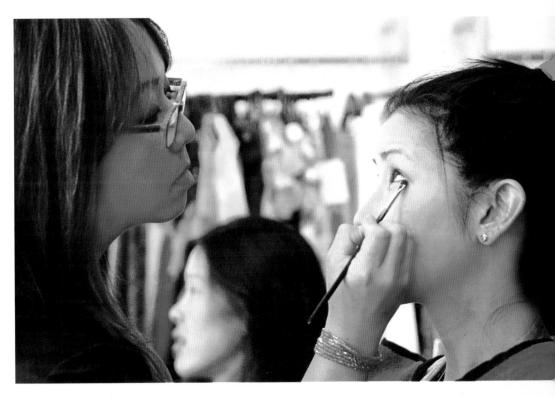

Making faces with Lisa Ling of *The View*.

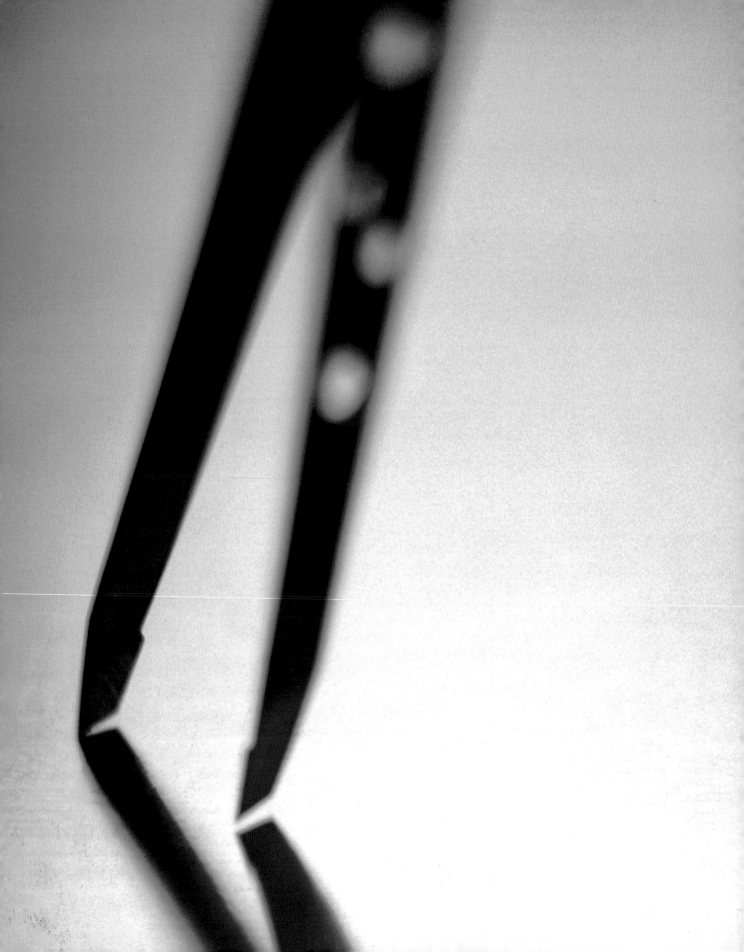

TOOLS OF
THE TRADE

1

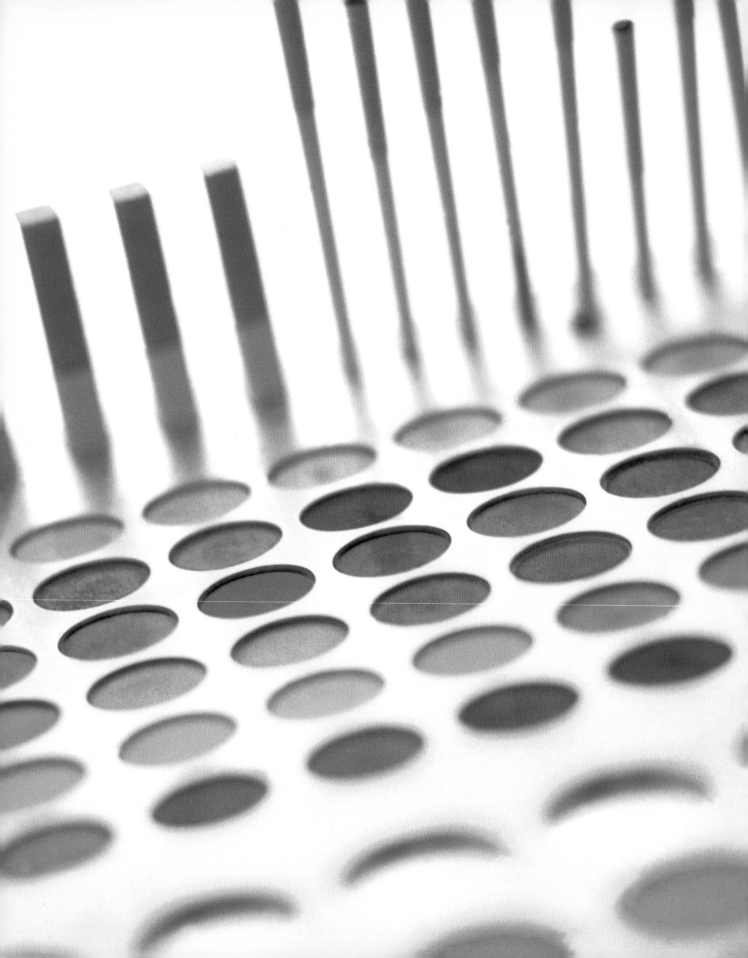

WHEN I WAS SIXTEEN, SOMEONE STOLE MY MAKEUP KIT. I WAS ABSOLUTELY DEVASTATED. TOOLS ARE TO A MAKEUP ARTIST WHAT A BRUSH IS TO A PAINTER, OR A SCALPEL TO A SURGEON. WITHOUT OUR KITS, WE CAN'T DO OUR JOB. I COULDN'T BEGIN TO IMAGINE HOW I WAS GOING TO REPLACE EVERYTHING. I WAS IN NEW YORK ON ASSIGNMENT AND WAS SUPPOSED TO HAVE DINNER WITH MY FRIEND THE ACTRESS ANDIE MCDOWELL. I HAD BEEN INTRODUCED TO HER THE YEAR BEFORE IN MILAN BY A CLOSE FRIEND SHE WAS DATING.

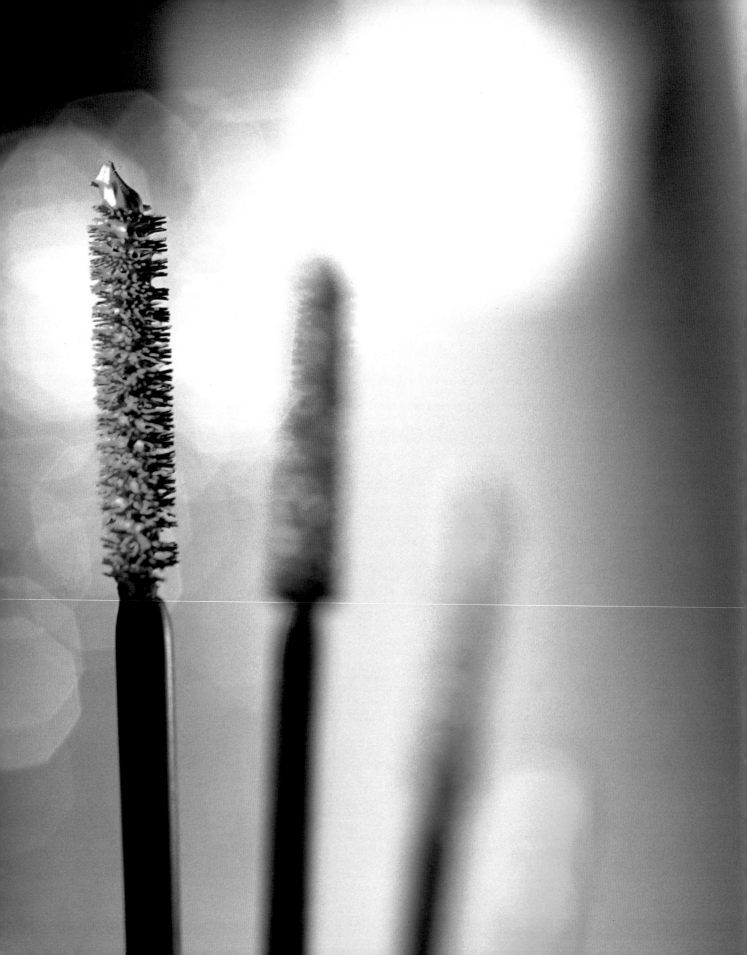

I'd moved there to do makeup when I was only fifteen, armed with a portfolio of work I'd been doing in Los Angeles all through high school.

On the night I was supposed to meet Andie for dinner, I was so upset that I called to cancel our plans. I just wanted to go home, but Andie insisted we spend the evening together. After dinner we went back to her apartment. Andie took me into the bedroom where she had a surprise for me—a brand-new makeup kit. It was an incredibly generous gesture, and one that I've never forgotten.

It goes without saying that professional makeup artists swear by their tools. Believe me, the right tools can make a huge difference in application, and you definitely don't want to cut corners. It's like buying a Yugo instead of a Mercedes. Which car do you think is the better ride? My advice: Buy the best. After all, good tools are an investment, and the results they deliver are incomparable.

There are dozens of different brushes on the market. If you can't afford them all, you'll need to invest in at least five of them: a blusher brush, a powder brush, a highlighter brush, a shadow brush, and an angled liner brush. In addition, you'll want to get a good pair of tweezers and an

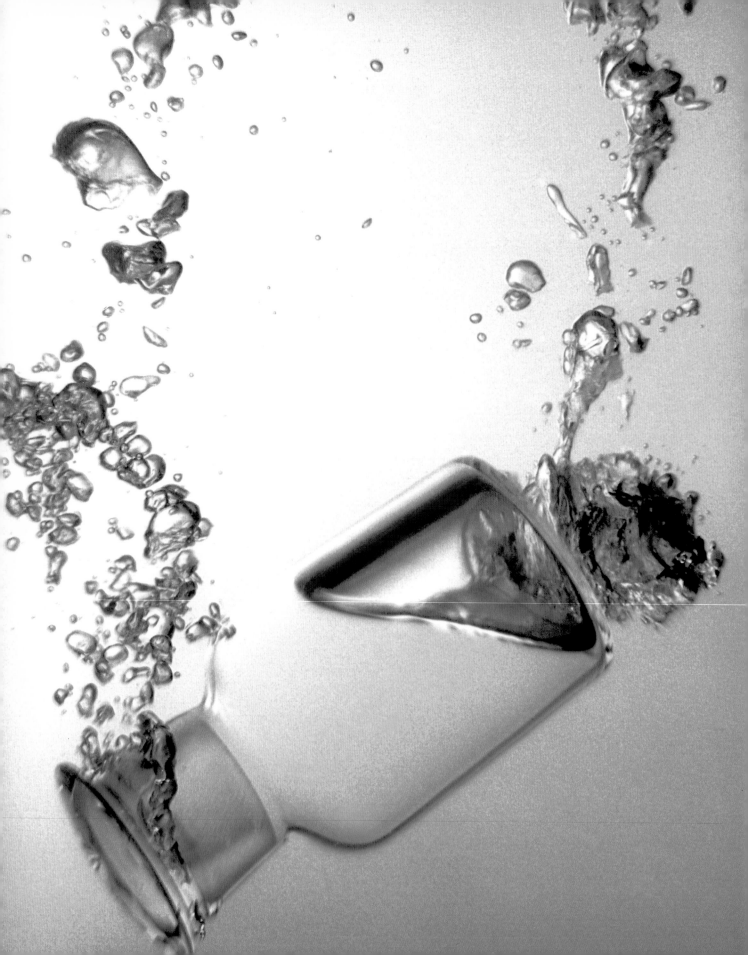

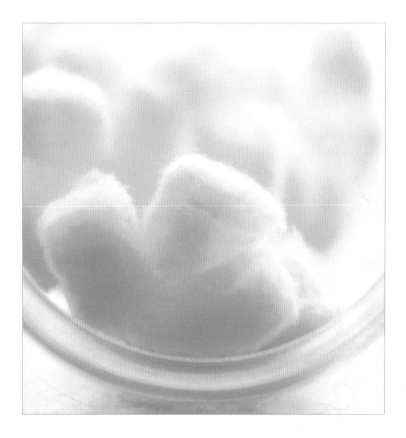

eyelash curler. Other essentials, like a powder puff and a set of latex sponges, are relatively inexpensive and should be replaced regularly.

Since Asian eyes tend to be small and have a flatter surface than most, it's a good idea to look for small, flat-head brushes to apply eye shadow.

What follows is a list of the tools that are always in my makeup kit. Refer to it when you're ready to start adding to your collection.

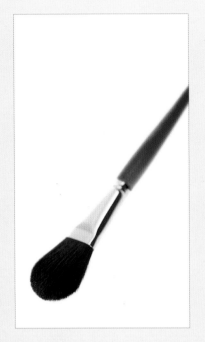
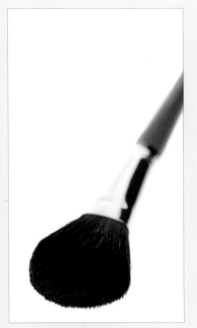
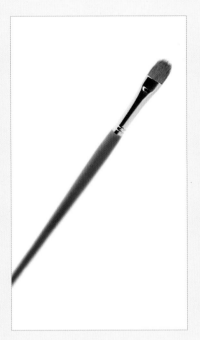

1

2

3

BLUSHER BRUSH

Tapered cut with a flat oval head to give the cheeks a healthy glow.

WHY YOU NEED IT

The denser bristles pick up a lot of product and allow you to deposit it precisely where you want it to go—say, on the apples of the cheeks. One of the most common mistakes women make when they're applying their own makeup is using the same brush to apply powder and blush. Blush should be applied to the cheekbones only. This is a relatively small area, perfect for a blusher brush with its medium round head and flat cut.

POWDER BRUSH

Larger and fuller than a blusher brush with a round head that allows you to apply loose powder over a large area.

WHY YOU NEED IT

The fluffy head picks up a light dusting of powder and distributes it evenly over the face. I use this brush constantly throughout the makeup application to reset powder and other makeup as it's applied.

FLAT-HEAD EYE SHADOW BRUSH

Small, dome-shaped, natural-hair brush for applying eye shadow.

WHY YOU NEED IT

The denser bristles and flat shape are perfect for depositing eye shadow directly to the eyelid just below the crease.

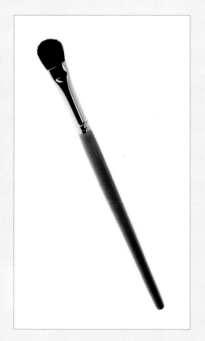
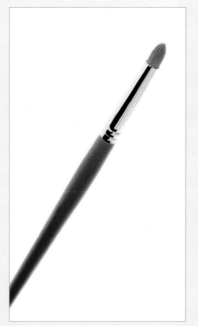
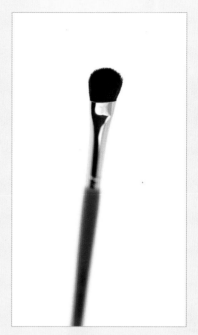

4

FULL-HEAD SHADOW BRUSH

Fluffy, dome-shaped brush for applying eye shadow all over the eyelid.

WHY YOU NEED IT

Covers a lot of territory in a hurry so it's perfect if you're using the same shade of shadow on the entire eyelid. But it also doubles as a highlighter brush or shadow blender brush.

5

CONTOUR CREASE BRUSH

Fluffy, tapered, natural-hair brush for adding depth and definition to the eyes.

WHY YOU NEED IT

Just the thing for Asian girls who want to create the illusion that their eyelids are not so flat. To give the eyes more depth, I use a darker shade of color on the lid and a highlighter under the brow bone. This brush lets you blend the shadow and highlighter together.

6

HIGHLIGHTER BRUSH

Fluffy, dome-shaped brush, slightly larger than the full-head shadow brush.

WHY YOU NEED IT

Again, this tool is perfect for Asian girls because it lets you create the illusion that your brow bone is a lot more prominent than it really is. Use it to apply highlighter directly underneath the brow bone to really open up your eyes.

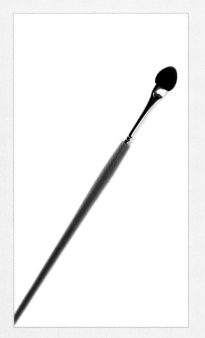
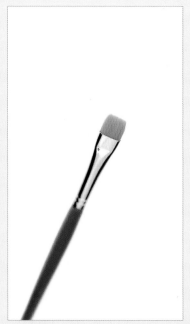
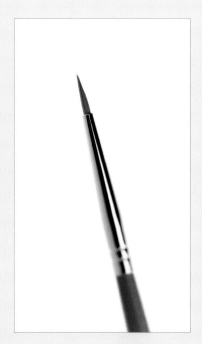

7

SPONGE-TIPPED APPLICATOR

Disposable multipurpose applicators that can last up to two months if cleaned properly.

WHY YOU NEED IT

Just the thing for applying cream eye shadow and smudging soft pencil eyeliner. These applicators are also terrific for blending eye shadows together, removing excess shadow if you get a little heavy-handed, and camouflaging blemishes or other minor skin imperfections—just dip the applicator into a little loose powder and dab it onto the area.

8

FLAT-HEAD BRUSH

Flat, synthetic bristles for applying cream eye shadows or concealers.

WHY YOU NEED IT

Great for getting concealer into hard-to-reach areas like under the eyelashes or in the crease of the nose. Also allows for a more even application of cream-based or wet powder eye shadow.

9

WET EYELINER BRUSH

Fine, pointy-tip brush for applying wet eyeliner.

WHY YOU NEED IT

The shape allows you to draw a precise line close to the lashes. Use it with liquid eyeliner or wet eye shadow. I love it for creating a hard-edged look in certain situations.

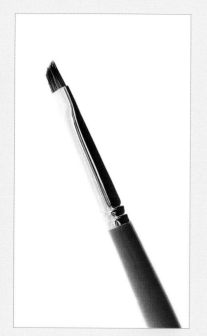
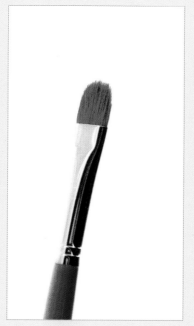

10

ANGLED LINER BRUSH
Soft yet firm natural bristles with an angled tip for lining the eyes.

WHY YOU NEED IT
The bristles are firm enough to pick up enough product to create a nice, smooth line close to the lashes. Use it with powder eye shadow only.

11

LIP BRUSH
Small, flat oval head and natural bristles for lip color and gloss.

WHY YOU NEED IT
Trust me, you just can't get lips to look as good without one. Use it to line the lips, then deposit color evenly.

12

LATEX SPONGE
Wedge-shaped synthetic sponge.

WHY YOU NEED IT
I couldn't live without my latex sponges, because they can be used in myriad ways: to apply foundation or concealer, to set powder underneath the eyes (the angle allows you to get close to the lash line) or in other tricky areas like around the hairline, to apply cheek gel, and to blend down heavily applied foundation, shadow, or cheek gel.

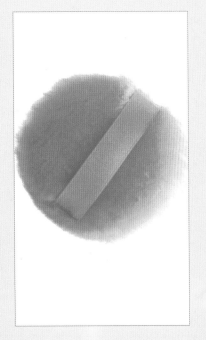

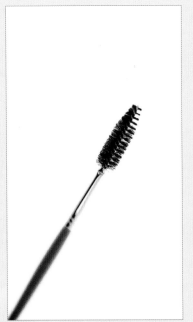

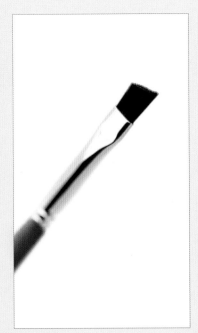

13

POWDER PUFF
Cotton puffs for loose or pressed powder.

WHY YOU NEED IT
The only tool you'll need to apply pressed powder. In a compact, they let you take the shine off your nose. I use them to set my loose powder. Think of it as literally pressing the powder into the skin. If you don't have a powder brush handy and want to use your loose powder, remember to shake the excess powder off the puff before using it on your face.

14

EYELASH GROOMING BRUSH
Resembles a mascara wand. Some have a plastic brush on one end to separate the lashes.

WHY YOU NEED IT
Use it to remove excess mascara after application.

15

ANGLED EYEBROW BRUSH
Hard synthetic bristles with an angled tip.

WHY YOU NEED IT
Can use it with pencils and powder shadows. If you have really thin brows, use a pencil first, then dip the eyebrow brush in a little powder shadow and go back over the brows.

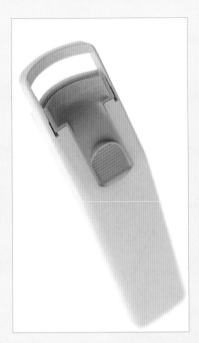

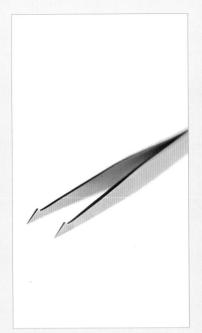

16

EYELASH CURLER

I prefer the new battery-operated models that heat up, because they hold the curl a bit longer than the conventional metal ones. The heat helps set the curl much as hot rollers would if you used them in your hair. They're also a lot gentler than metal eyelash curlers, because they work so quickly.

WHY YOU NEED IT

Great for Asian girls because our lashes are so hard to curl.

17

TWEEZERS

Angle-tipped, pointy-tipped, and flat-head.

WHY YOU NEED THEM

You'll need a pair of pointy-tipped tweezers for individual or ingrown hairs and a pair of angle-tipped or flat-head tweezers for regular plucking. Choose stainless steel tweezers that won't rust or corrode. Mehaz makes a variety of models, including the Rubis tweezers, which can grasp even the finest hairs.

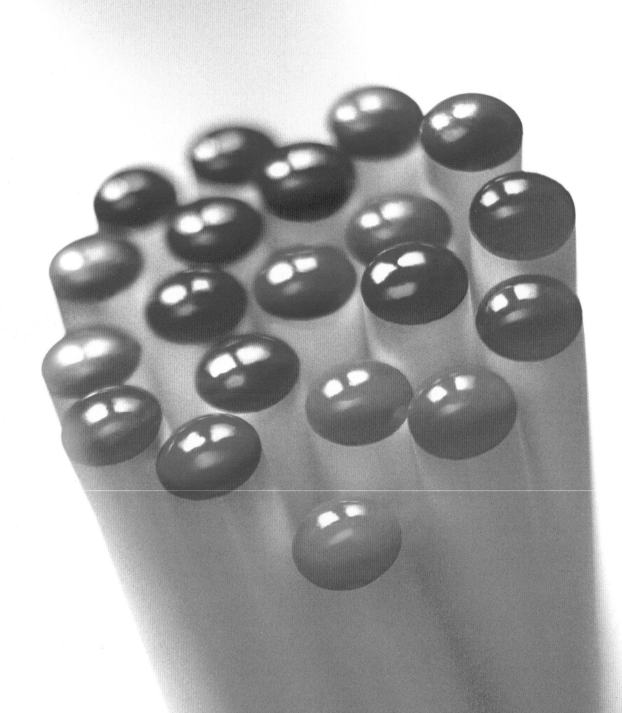

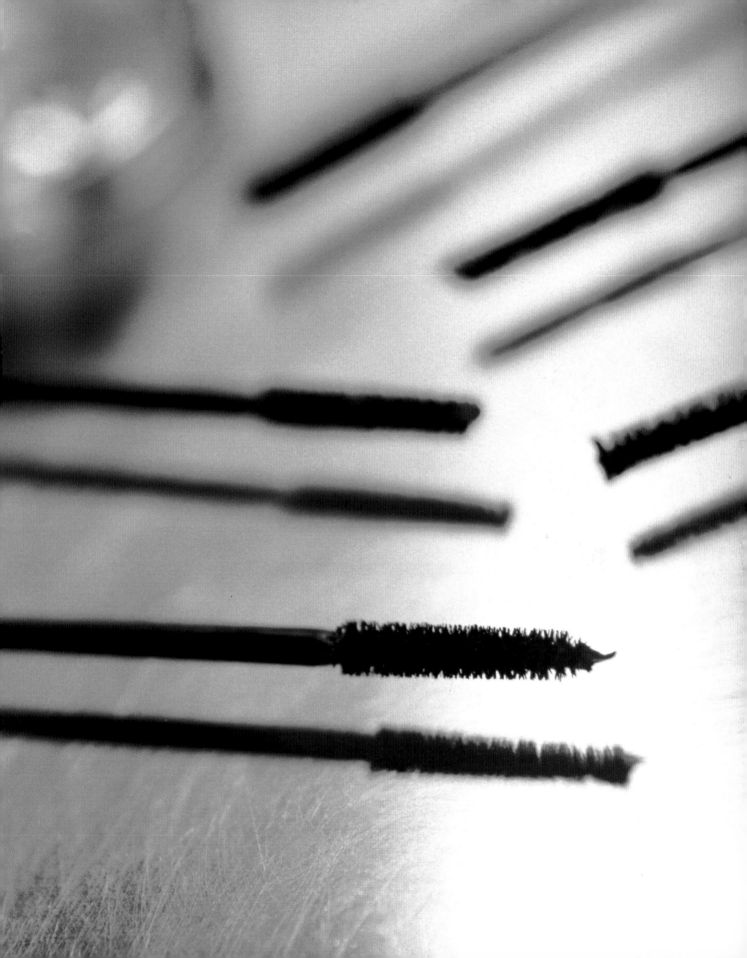

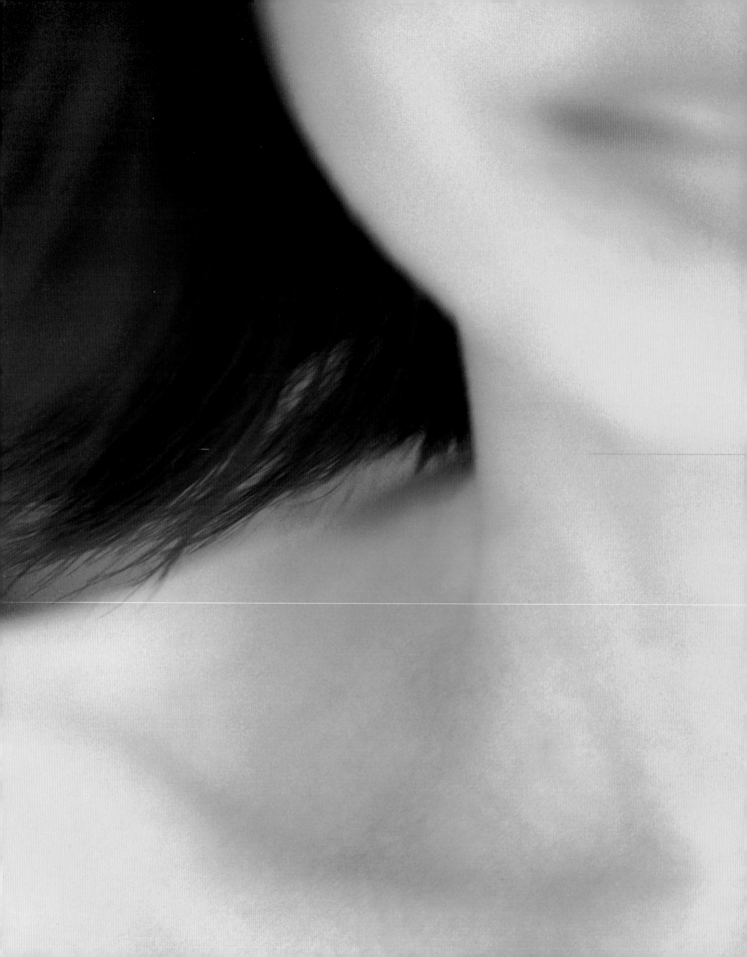

TRICKS OF THE TRADE

✳ Use a flat-tipped brush instead of your fingertip to apply concealer. You'll get a lot more control that way.

✳ Use a brush and powder instead of a pencil to line your eyes. It gives a softer look, plus there's less tendency to stretch and pull the delicate skin around the eye, which tends to lose collagen as we age. Powders also give you the option of creating smoky eyes that don't look so hard and edgy.

✳ Keep your reusable sponges clean by washing them with mild soap and water, then air-drying them completely.

✳ Do not use samples or testers at the beauty counter. Ask for a clean, unused applicator and apply makeup to your hand, not your face. One department store that tested its samples discovered that 5 percent of testers were infected with fungus and other contaminants.

✳ Check your makeup bag every month and discard any makeup that has a rancid smell or has lost its consistency.

✳ Try being creative with your brushes. For example, use a lip brush instead of a shadow brush to apply glitter around the eyes. The idea is to be as precise as possible, which is why a lip brush makes sense. The shape—small and pointy—is perfect for getting into tight spaces.

✳ Wash your hands and face before applying makeup.

✳ Wipe your makeup bottles, jars, and tubes with disinfectant if they become dirty or dusty.

✳ Discard eye cosmetics after six months, mascara after three.

✳ Take good care of your brushes. Wash natural-hair brushes in a gentle shampoo and warm water at least twice a month. There's no need to soak your brushes. Simply wet them under the tap, pour a little shampoo into the palm of your hand, and swish the brushes around in the lather. Rinse well and smooth out the bristles with your fingers. Let the brushes air-dry on a clean towel.

THINGS TO KEEP IN YOUR PURSE

A compact, lipstick or lip gloss, mascara, and blush are all you need to "put a face together" anywhere, anytime.

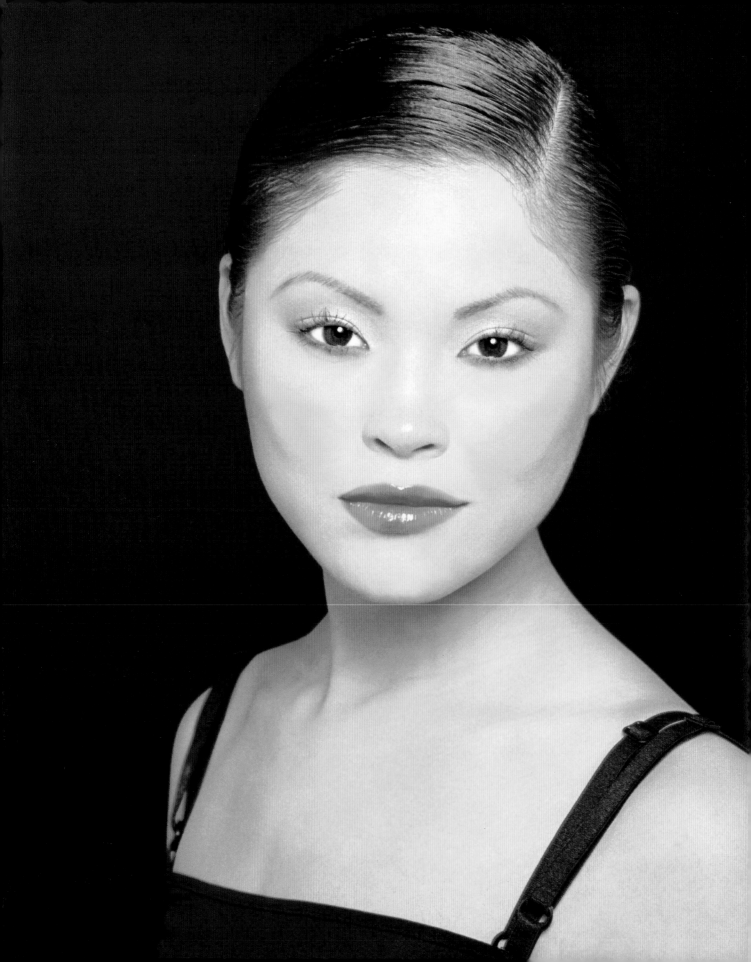

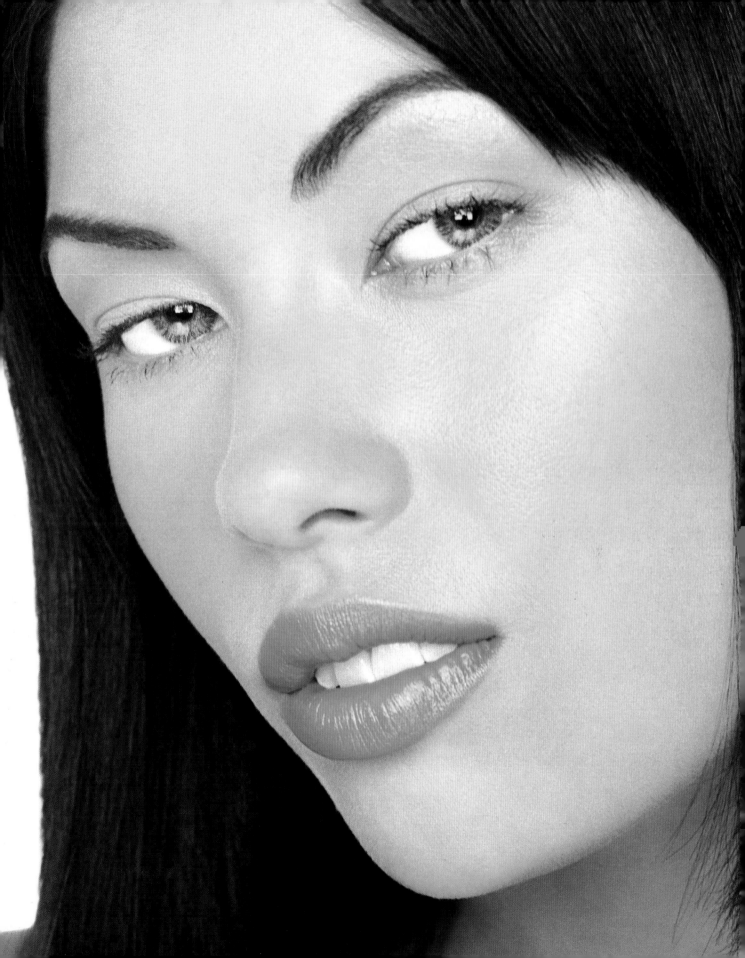

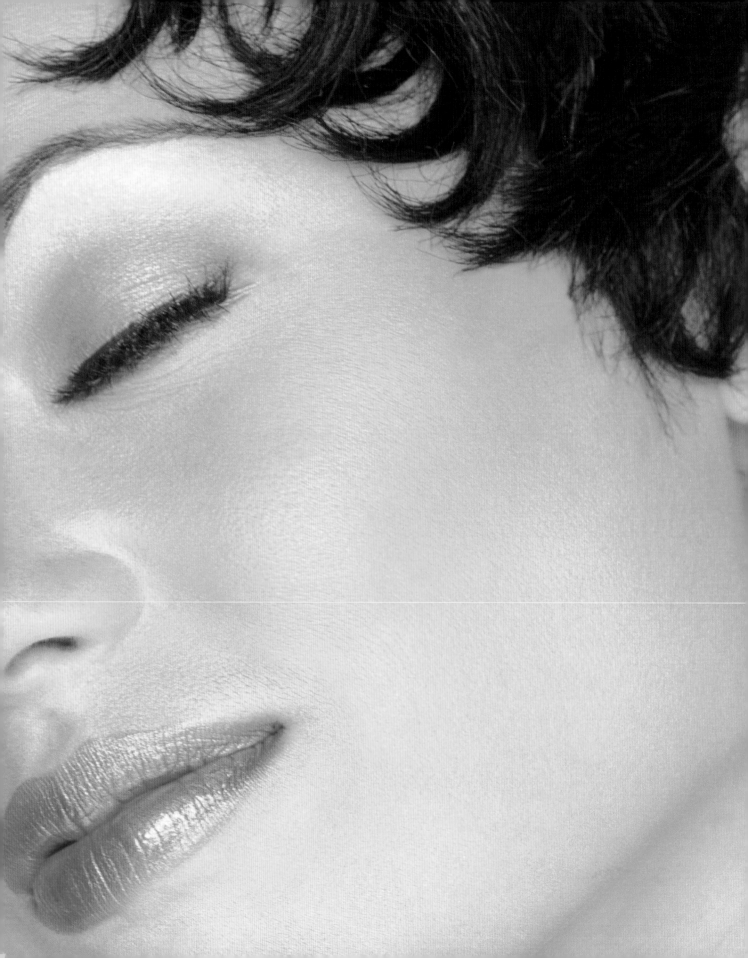

2

TRADE SECRETS

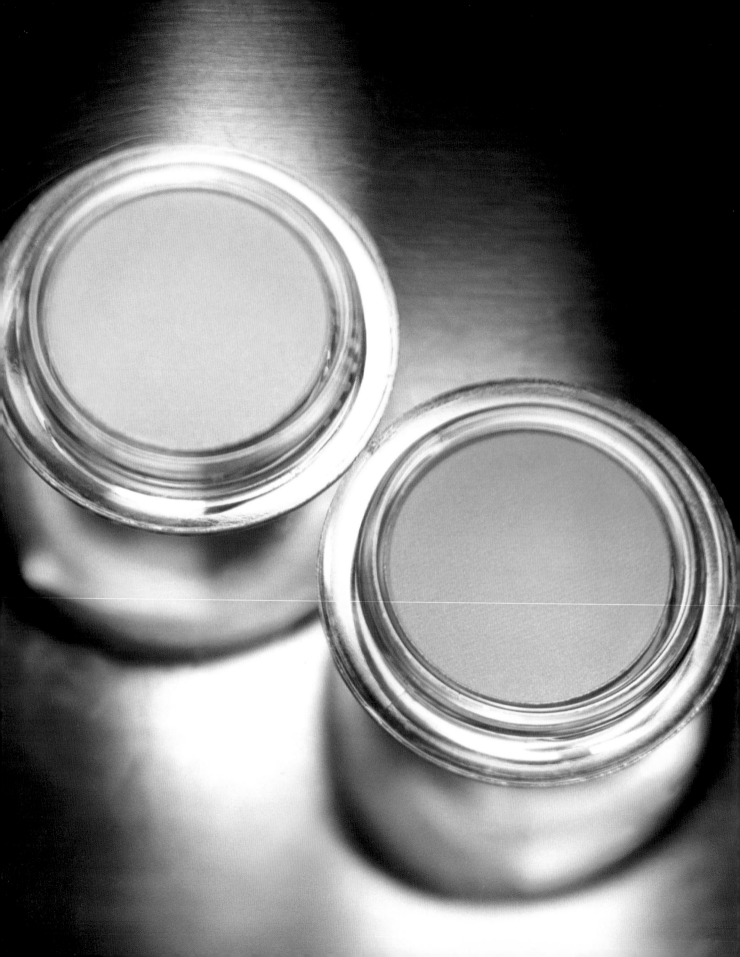

WHEN I WORKED ON THE FILM *RANSOM* WITH MEL GIBSON, WE WENT ON LOCATION TO AN AIRPLANE HANGAR WHERE WE HAD TO USE ONE OF THE OFFICES TO DO HAIR AND MAKEUP. I HAD JUST GIVEN MEL A HAIRCUT, AND WE WERE KIND OF KICKING BACK AND KIDDING AROUND WITH THE DIRECTOR, RON HOWARD, WHEN WE NOTICED THAT THERE WAS A PRETTY LITTLE GIRL WATCHING US FROM THE DOOR-WAY. MEL INVITED HER TO JOIN US. AFTER WE'D ALL BEEN TALKING FOR A WHILE, SHE ASKED US HOW WE GOT SO SUCCESSFUL, MEL AS AN ACTOR, and me as a makeup artist. Neither of us knew quite what to say. Finally Mel looked at me and said, "That must be one of the hardest questions to answer."

I think we ended up telling her that it was probably a combination of luck and being at the right place at the right time. But it got me thinking: there's probably a little more to it than that. Maybe it's because I've never set limits for myself. I'm self-taught, so I've always made my own rules instead of following someone else's. Maybe it's because I had to deal with issues of beauty when I was a teenager, and so I learned very early how to bring out the best in everyone I work with. A lot of it has to do with pure instinct, simply knowing what looks good and what doesn't. When someone sits in my chair without any makeup on, I can visualize exactly how she or he will look when I'm done.

My approach to makeup is very clean and blended. I'm not one for using heavy powders, shadows, or liners that tend to lie on the surface of the skin. That's probably why I've had such an extensive clientele of male celebrities. I know how to cover their flaws without covering up who they are.

I am probably the queen of blending. In fact, I don't think it's possible to overblend. The more you work the colors into the skin where they'll mix with your own oils, the more natural your makeup will look. Blending also sets your makeup so you'll look flawless all day.

Over the years I've developed a few techniques that contribute to my signature style. By the time you've finished reading this book, you should have a clear understanding of how to use these techniques to create a look that works for you.

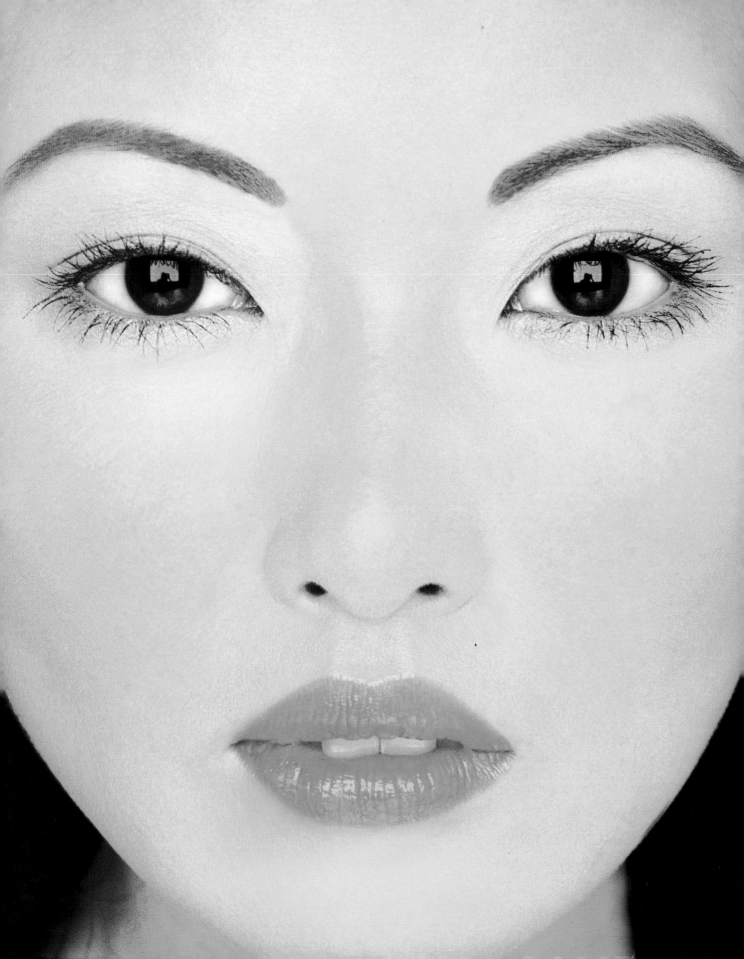

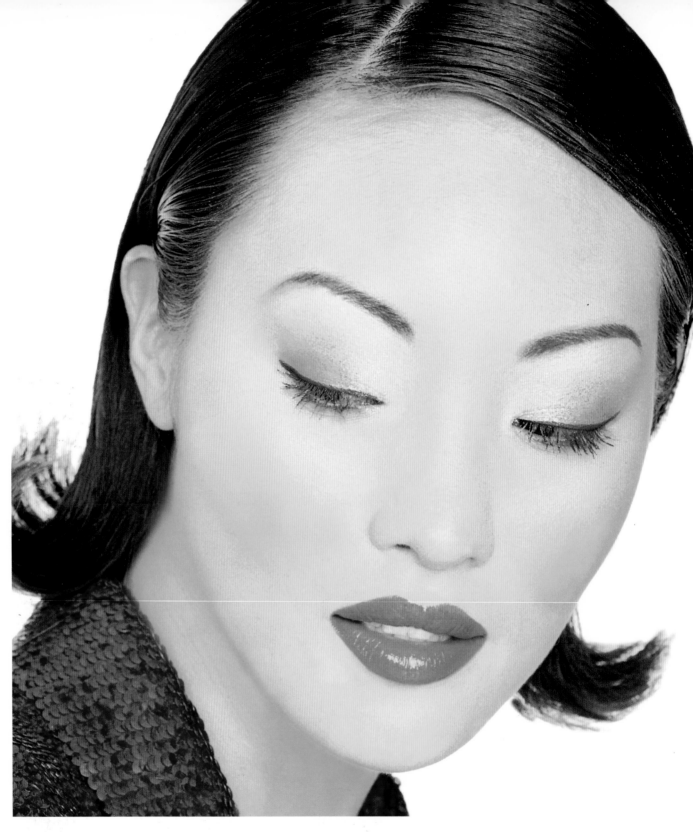

Use the Shadows and Light technique with shimmery shades of eye shadow to create a theatrical look. Here I applied highlighter on the inner part of the lid and a dramatic shade of eye shadow on the outer part.

SHADOWS AND LIGHT

The Shadows and Light technique allows you to play up your best features and camouflage your flaws. It's all about creating illusions. Objects recede into the darkness but become more prominent when placed in the light. By applying those same principles to makeup, I am able to work the same magic. I use highlights to lift and enhance certain features and darker colors to do just the opposite. Working with shadows and light on an Asian canvas enables us to wear the same colors as women of other ethnicities; we just have to wear them differently.

For example, Asian eyes tend to be small and close-set, yet many Asian women want their eyes to look bigger and farther apart. By using a highlighter on the brow bone and a lighter shade of eye shadow at the inner corner of the eye, you'll create the illusion that your eyes are bigger and farther apart.

By applying dark eye shadow in the crease of the eyelid, you'll actually create the illusion of a fold there.

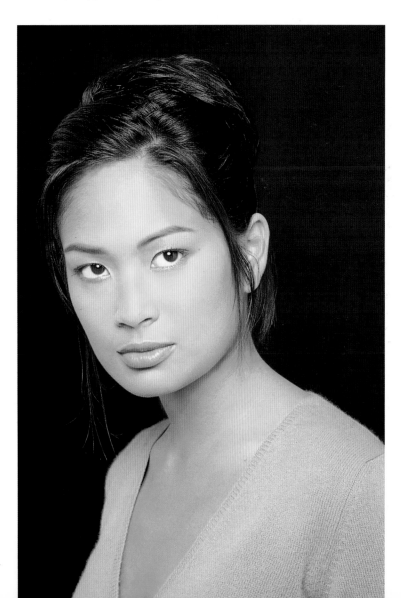

The look here is subtle, yet sophisticated. The trick is to work with neutral colors and soft shades of beige, nutmeg, and rose. Again, I used the lighter shades on the inner part of the lid and the deeper shades on the outer part of the lid.

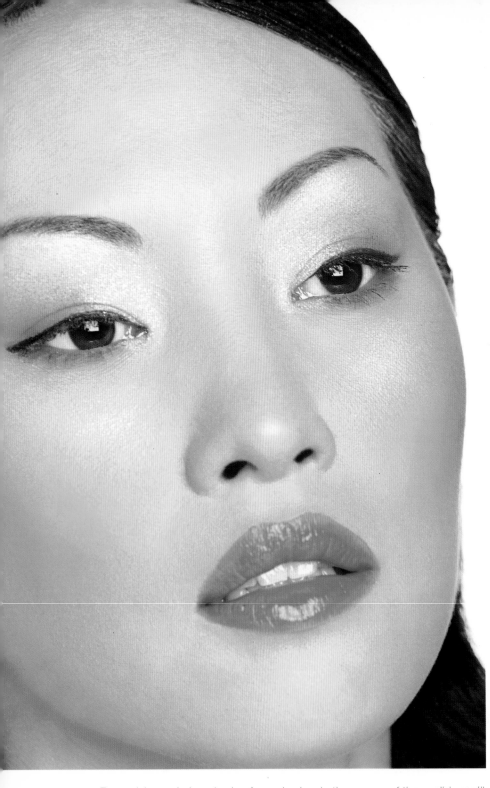

Women with round faces who weren't blessed with really great cheekbones can fake them with the Shadows and Light technique. Just use a highlighter color on the top part of the apples of the cheeks and a darker shade of blush on the lower part of the apples. Blend the two shades together and you've got instant cheekbones.

By applying a darker shade of eye shadow in the crease of the eyelid, you'll actually create the illusion of a fold there.

Or let's say you feel that the bridge of your nose is too flat. Use your finger to run a little highlighter powder along the bridge of your nose, then brush some translucent powder over it to define that area. It's the same principle: objects that are placed in the light appear more prominent.

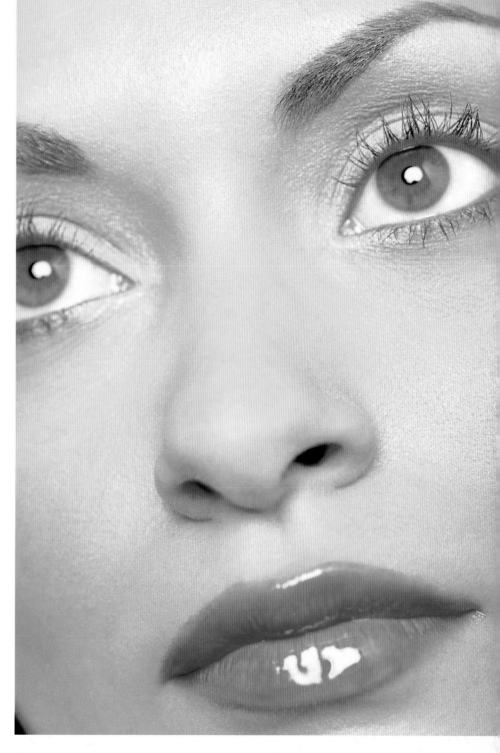

To emphasize the brow bone, apply a lighter shade of eye shadow there.

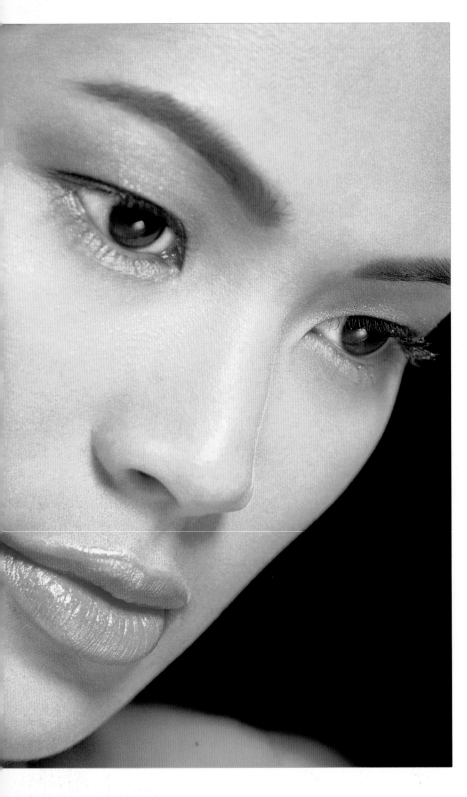

I have always found that regardless of our differences, all Asian faces have one thing in common—they're very mysterious. Working with shadows and light allows us to retain that sense of mystery, not obliterate it. By using Shadows and Light technique effectively, you'll still look Asian while enhancing your unique features.

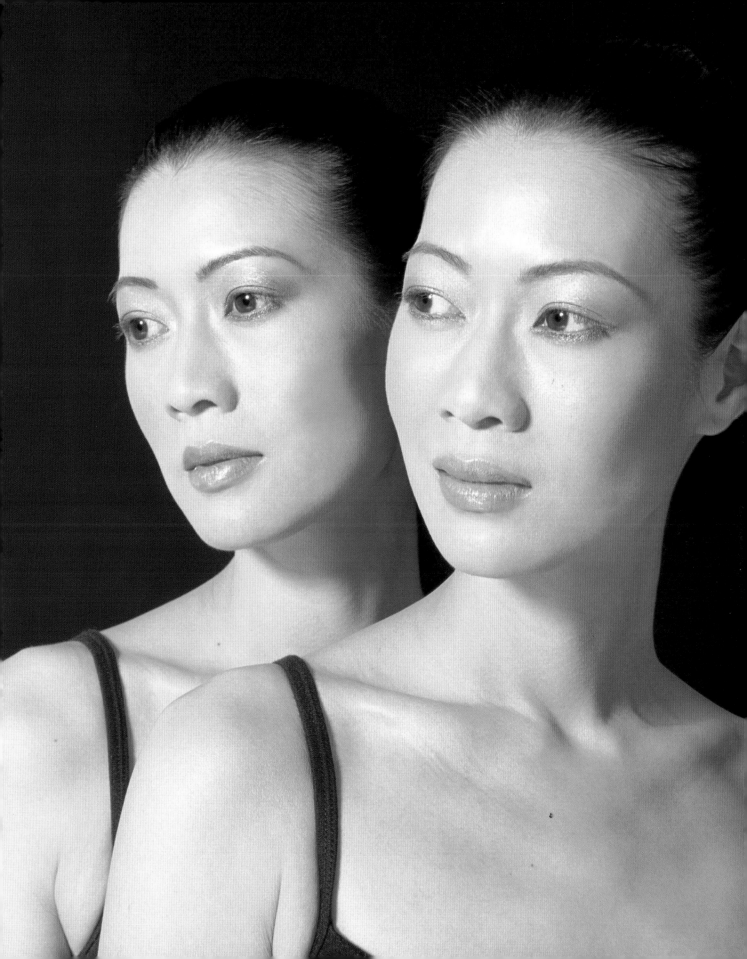

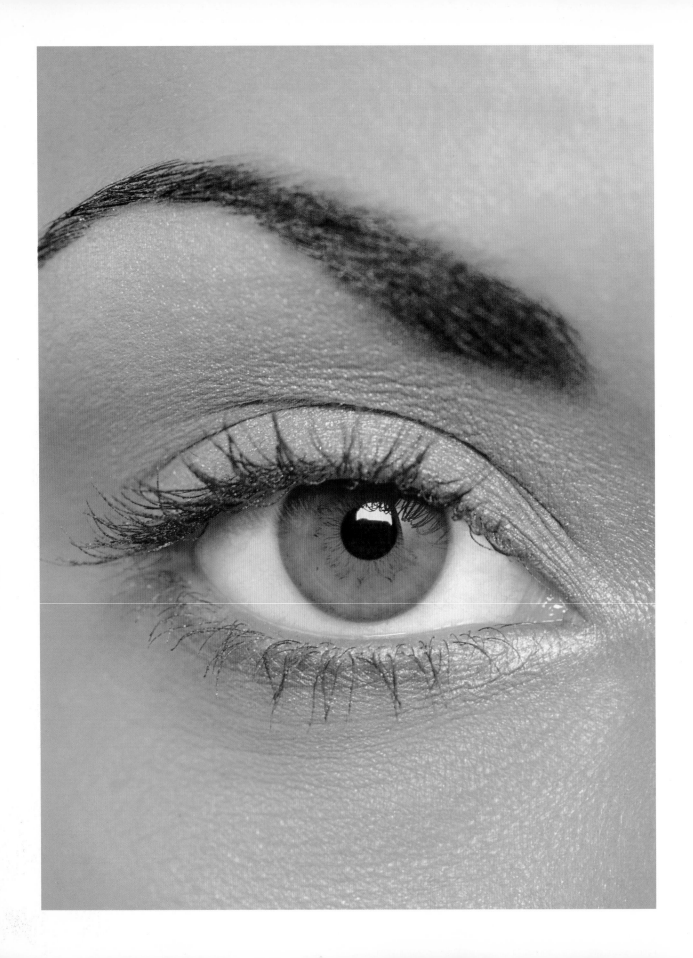

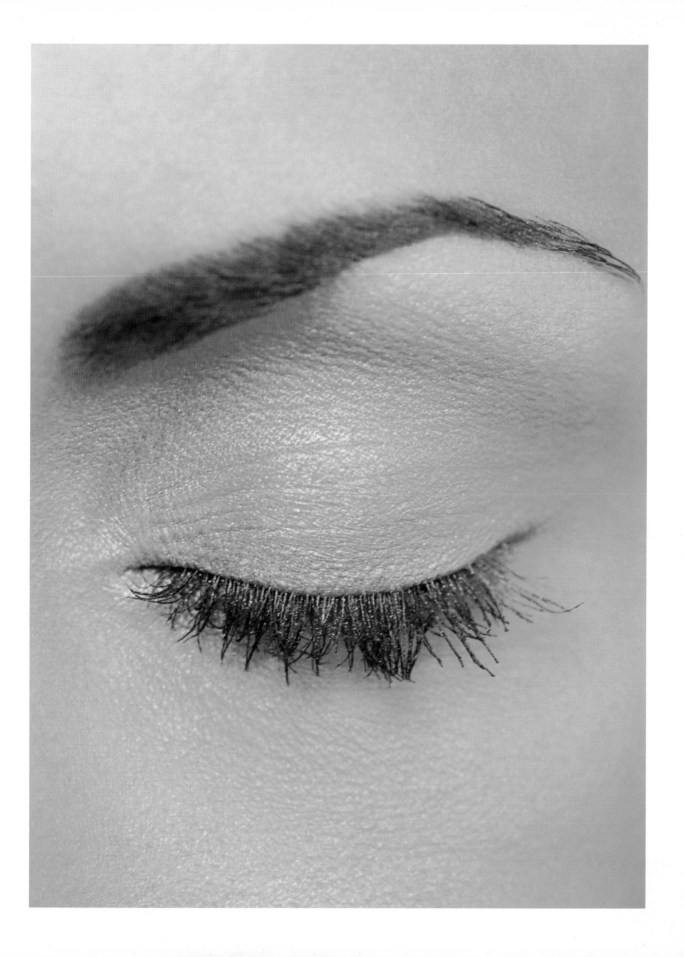

BLENDING

I cannot stress enough the importance of blending. After all, you don't want to look like your makeup is wearing you. If you take the time to blend everything carefully, you won't.

Blending becomes really essential when working with eye shadow. The trick is to blend the colors into the skin so well that they seem to become part of who you are instead of just sitting on the surface of the skin.

One thing you'll need is a good set of blending brushes. I use a mini–blusher brush to go over the eyes once I've got the shadow on. It allows me to remove the excess shadow and blend all the colors together.

Blending is crucial when it comes to applying foundation. You don't want to stop at the jawline. Instead, blend foundation all the way down the neck to avoid a noticeable line of demarcation. Also, make sure to blend it into the hairline. Don't forget the ears, especially if they're a different shade from your face and neck.

1

2

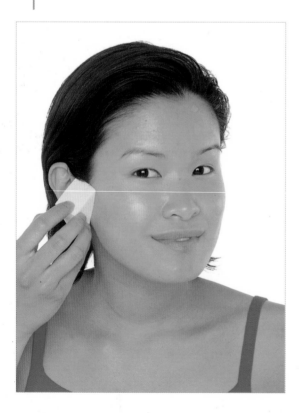

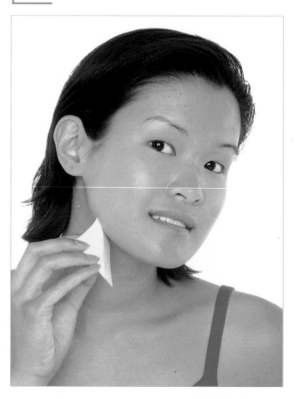

It's important to blend foundation into the hairline.

Take the time to blend foundation all the way down the neck to avoid any line of demarcation.

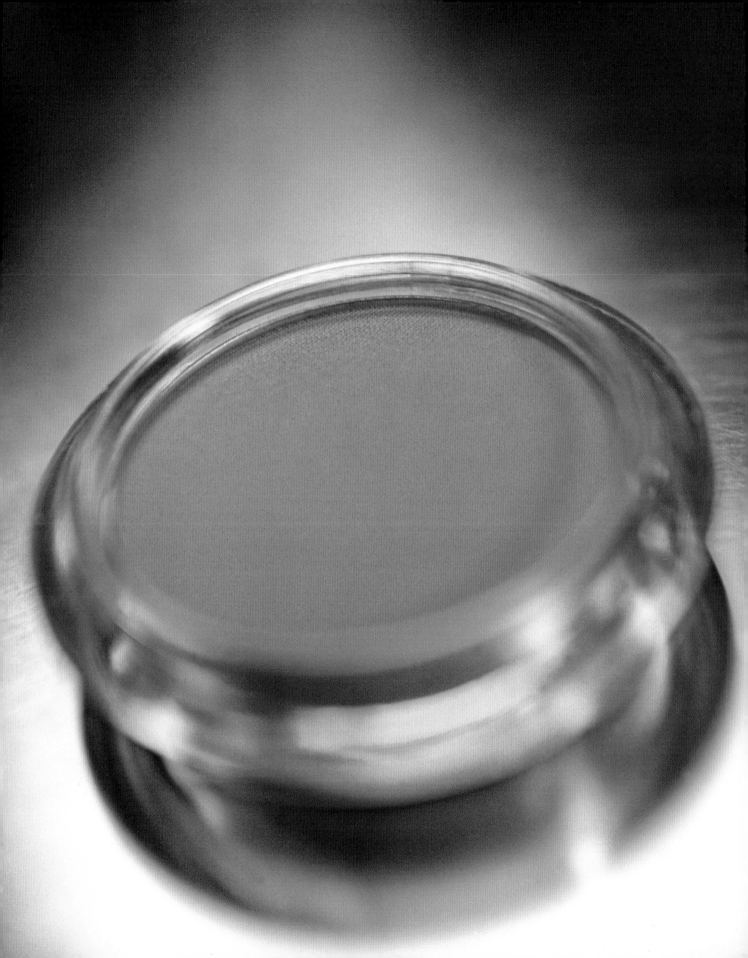

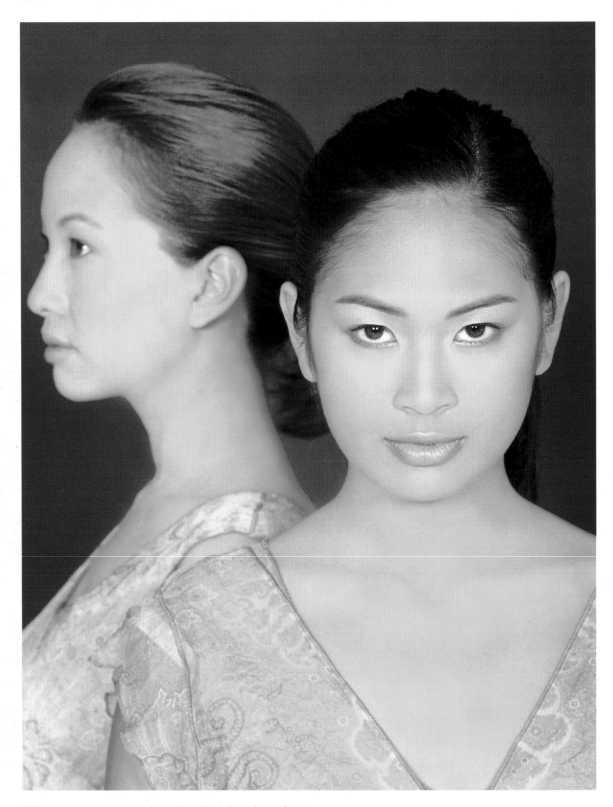

Blending is the key to a face that doesn't look made up.

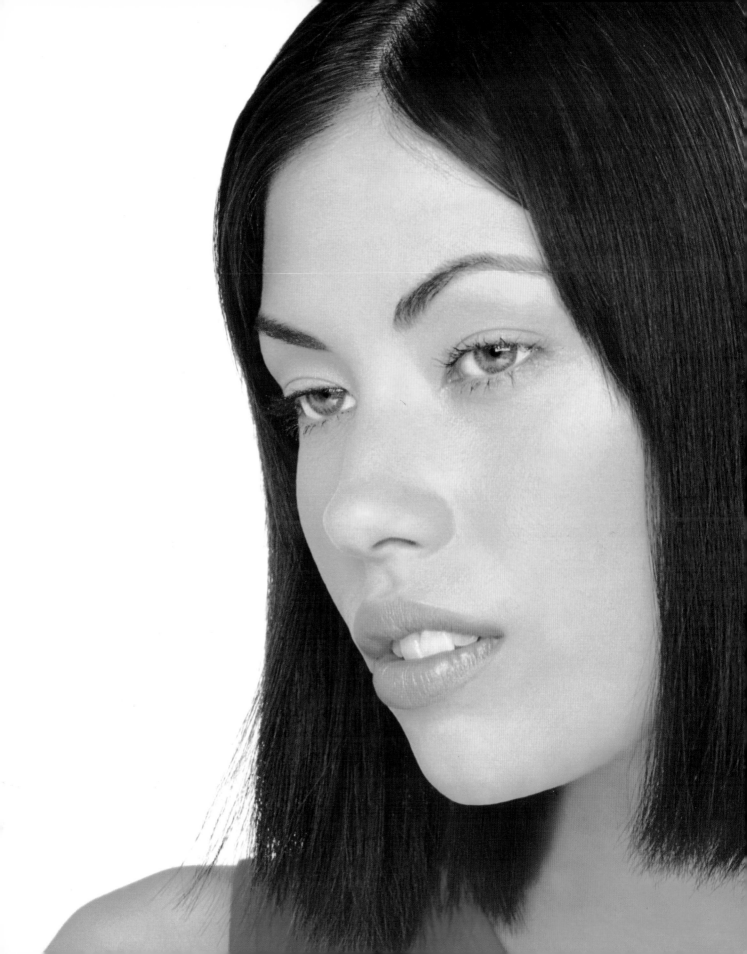

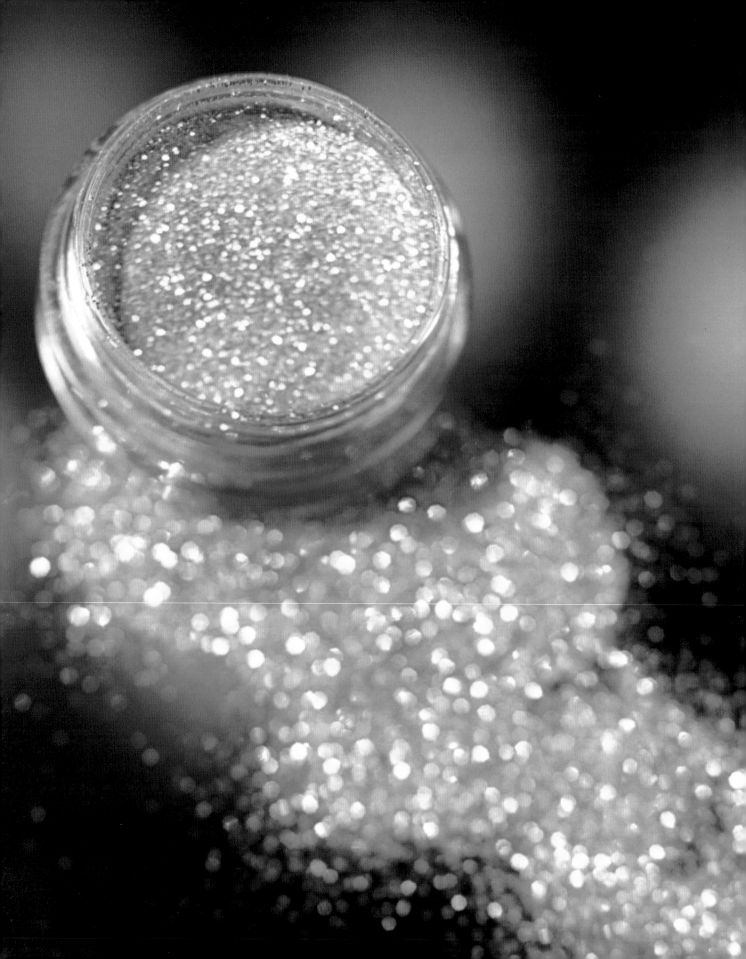

SPARKLE AND SHIMMER

You can add a little sparkle and shimmer to your look by learning how to use iridescent loose powders or glitter, which is coarser, shinier, and more reflective (it's like adding little jewels to the face).

Essentially pure pigment, shimmery powders were created for use by professionals who wanted to enhance eye shadows or lipstick. It's a very dramatic look, but don't be afraid to experiment with it. For instance, if you mix a shimmery pure pigment with clear lip gloss, you can create a whole new product.

I like to use the Shadows and Light technique with Sparkle and Shimmer. Just use a lighter shade of iridescent powder on the areas you want to highlight and a darker shade on those you don't.

A classic Sparkle and Shimmer look with lots of warmth. Note the glitter on the lids, the lip gloss mixed with gold dust, even the shimmer powder mixed with translucent powder on the cheeks.

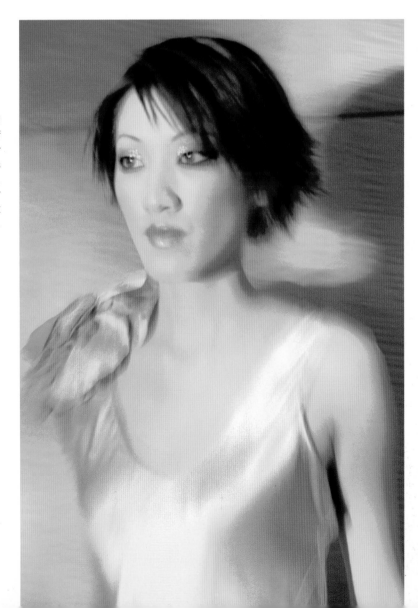

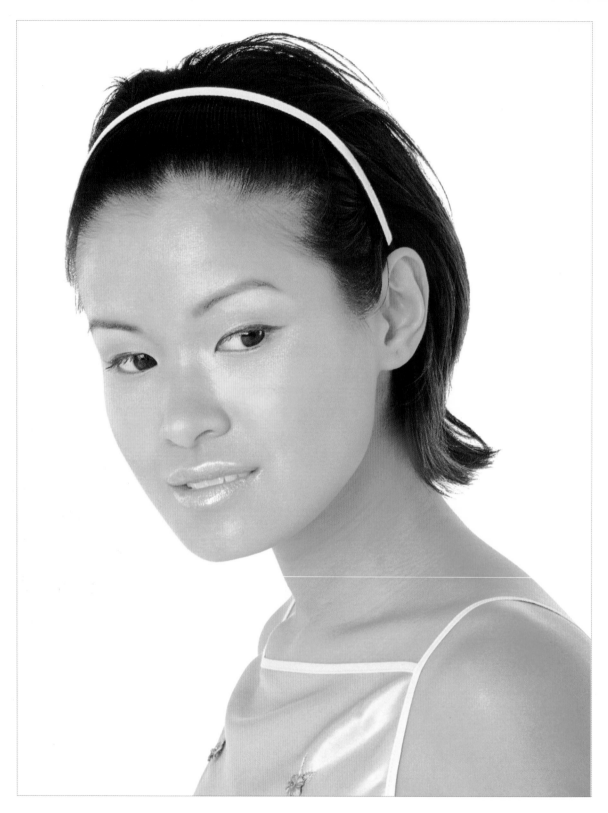

Turn down the volume on the Sparkle and Shimmer technique by using softer shades of shimmery shadow and staying away from the glitter. Here I used pale shades of pink, blue, and silver to create a cool, ice-princess look.

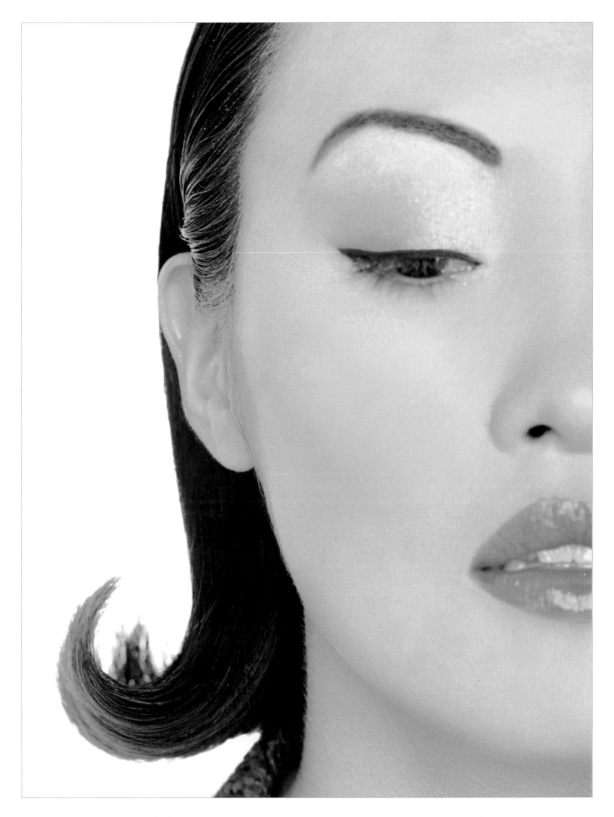

Here I used pearl-colored glitter on the inner part of the lid and soft pearlized dust on the brow bone. I also applied red glitter on the middle to outer lid. Lip gloss mixed with pure pigment provided the finishing touch.

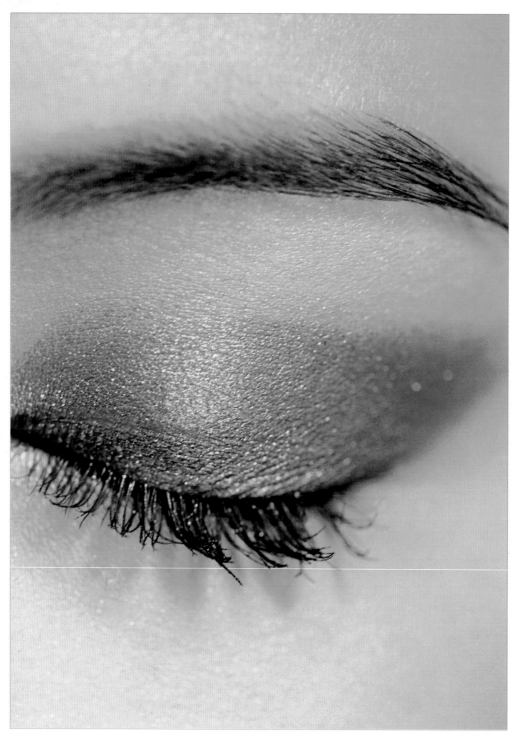

For more depth and intensity, apply your shimmery eye shadow wet.

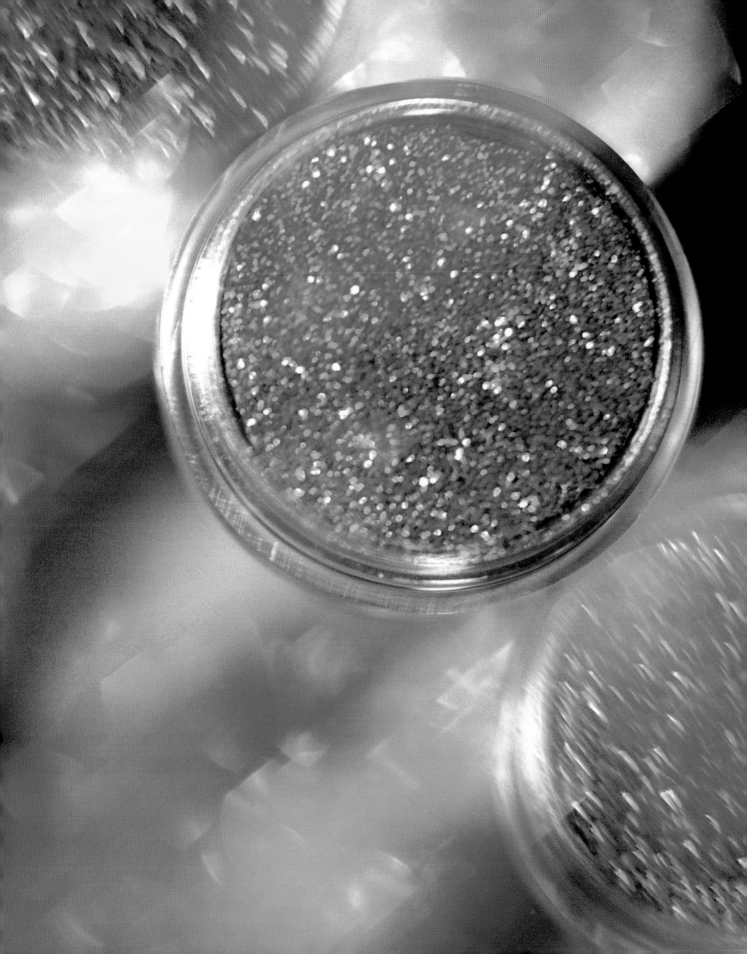

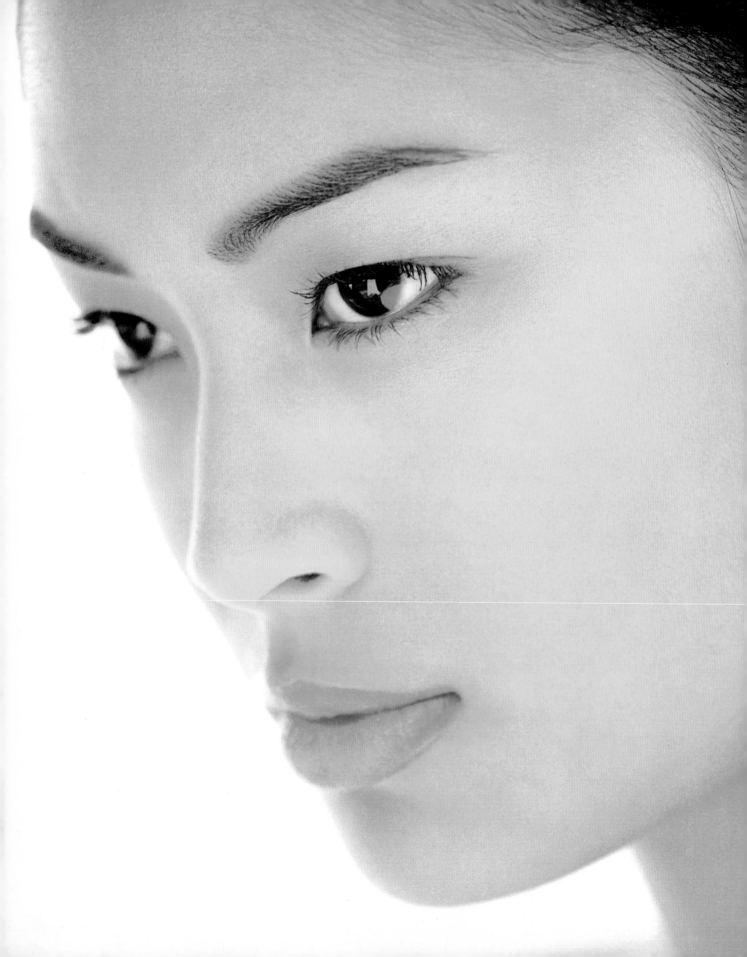

3
SKIN-DEEP

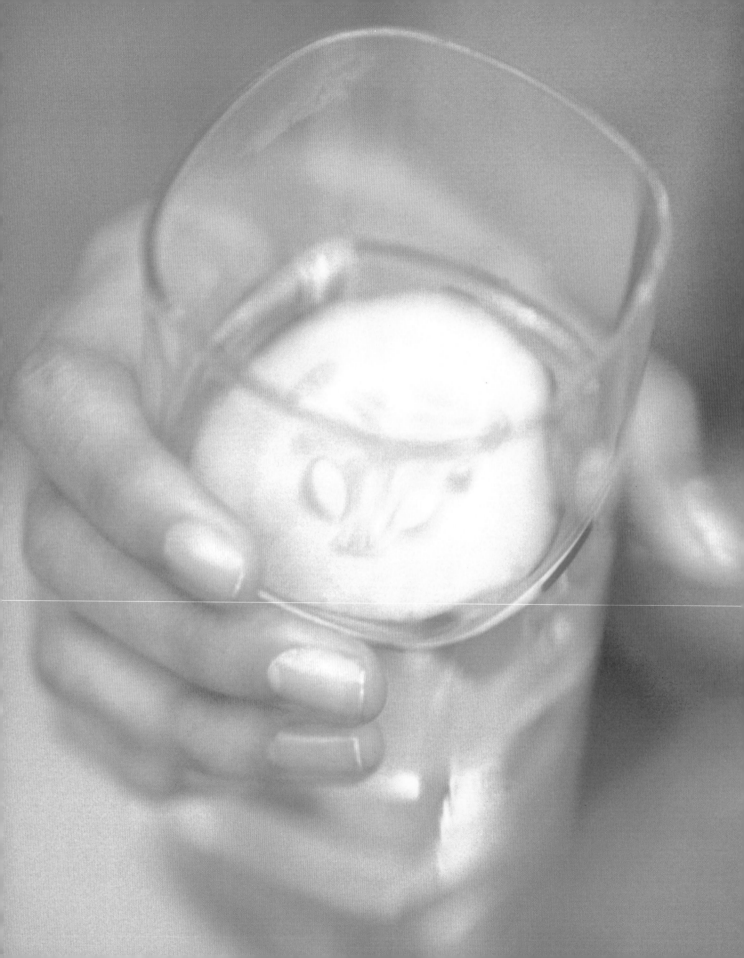

THERE'S NOTHING A MAKEUP ARTIST LIKES BETTER THAN TO WORK ON A CLEAR, RADIANT COMPLEXION. HEALTHY-LOOKING SKIN JUST GLOWS, AND IT MAKES OUR WORK LOOK THAT MUCH BETTER. AFTER ALL, A SMOOTHER CANVAS MAKES FOR A PRETTIER PICTURE. FORTUNATELY, MOST ASIAN WOMEN ARE BLESSED WITH GOOD SKIN, BUT IT TENDS TO BE DELICATE, WHICH IS WHY IT'S IMPORTANT TO WEAR SUNSCREEN EVERY DAY. IT'S ALSO A GOOD IDEA TO DEVELOP A SKIN-CARE REGIMEN THAT WORKS FOR YOU AND STICK TO IT. BUT REMEMBER, your skin reflects what's going on inside your body, which is why it's essential to get

enough rest, drink plenty of water, exercise regularly, watch what you eat, and find ways

to reduce stress in your life. If you don't, you'll pay the price in the form of everything from

blemishes to dark circles under the eyes.

I take very good care of my skin. For one thing, I use only high-quality products—

cleansers, toners, moisturizers, a gentle exfoliant once a week, and an at-home mask.

I also think it's important to switch formulations depending on the season. In the winter,

for example, when central heating can deplete your skin of precious moisture, you might

need a heavier, more emollient moisturizer, but you'll probably want something lighter in

the summertime. I'm also a big fan of eye creams, which are formulated specifically for

delicate skin around the eyes. Sunscreen is important too, especially when you live in

California like I do. I also try to drink lots of water, get plenty of rest, and wash my face

every night before going to bed, no matter how tired I am or how late it is. But if I do have

a breakout, there's nothing like a good sweat at the gym for releasing toxins. My thing is

running. I love the way my skin looks after a vigorous run or a really hard workout. It just

glows.

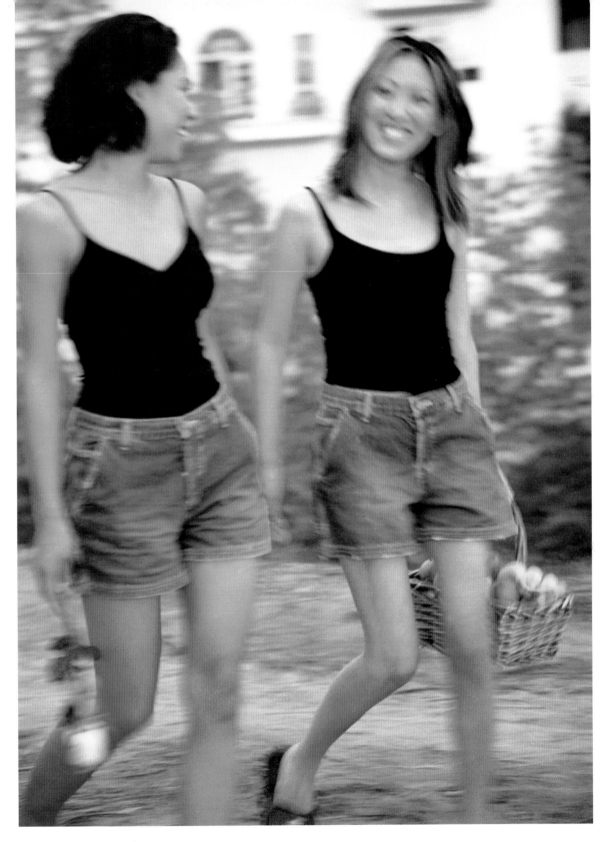

Taking a walk with a friend is a good way to relieve stress, which can do wonders for your complexion.

ABOUT FACE

If you have a serious acne condition, it's best to see a dermatologist, but for routine maintenance there's nothing like regular facials. I have one every four weeks with Cornelia Zicu, an esthetician at the Peninsula Spa in New York City. Think of it as visiting your dental hygienist for a thorough cleaning that goes way beyond what regular brushing and flossing can do. Our cells may start out plump and juicy (they actually regenerate every twenty-eight days), but once they sit on the surface for any length of time, the skin can look dull. That's where an esthetician comes in.

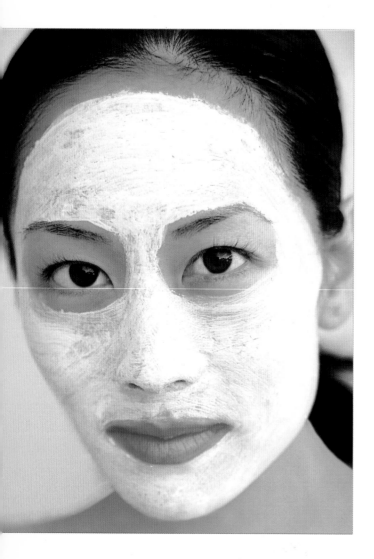

First she'll steam your face to stimulate circulation and make it easier to perform extractions, unclogging the pores and removing blackheads and other debris that can make the skin look uneven. But the best part of the facial has to be the massage. Not only does it feel wonderful, it stimulates the circulation, accelerating the skin's natural ability to rid itself of impurities. Massage also encourages lymph drainage, eliminating toxins—everything from makeup to pollution and cigarette smoke. Better yet, it stimulates the production of collagen and elastin, keeping wrinkles at bay and helping the skin look firmer. Your esthetician can customize an agenda for you, recommending products specifically for your skin type.

Use a mask designed for your skin type at least once a week.

MOISTURIZE

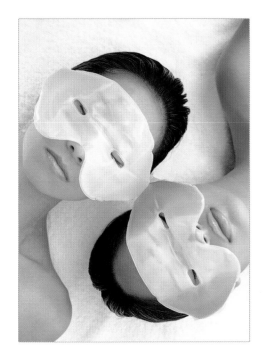

Moisturizers as we know them have been based on the Galenic formula since 500 B.C., when a Greek named Galen found a way to combine beeswax and borax to keep the skin from losing moisture, literally sealing it in. But as Rebecca James Gadberry, instructor of Cosmetic Sciences at UCLA Extension, Los Angeles, points out, science is changing the way moisturizers work. "New technology enables us to load moisturizers up with high-performance ingredients that create activity inside the skin," she says. "You're not just creating a barrier."

Skin-care companies started adding vitamins A, C, and E (the antioxidants) to their products when it was discovered that they may guard against the damaging effects of sun, smoking, and other environmental factors. Some products may actually help the skin rehydrate itself.

Helen Famularé, spa-training manager/ skin-care specialist at the Elizabeth Arden Red Door Salon and Spa in New York City, finds that Asian women in general tend to overdo it when it comes to moisturizers, which can clog the pores. Her advice: easy does it. "You don't need heavy creams with a lot of oils," she says. "You're better off using a ceramide capsule and a light moisturizer with an SPF 15."

Reduce puffiness by wearing a chilled eye mask or placing cucumber slices on the eyes.

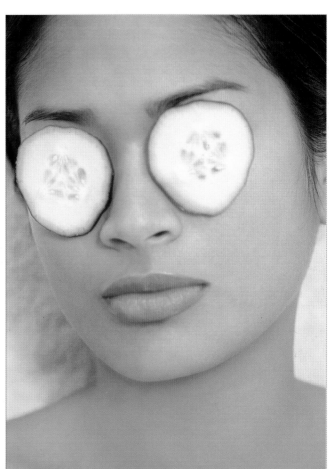

GET EVEN

The key to a flawless complexion is regular exfoliation, which sloughs off dead skin cells and leaves the complexion looking radiant. There are a number of products you can use at home once a week, including fruit enzymes, fruit acids, and scrubs containing gentle exfoliants like oatmeal or cornmeal. Avoid almond scrubs, which can be too abrasive.

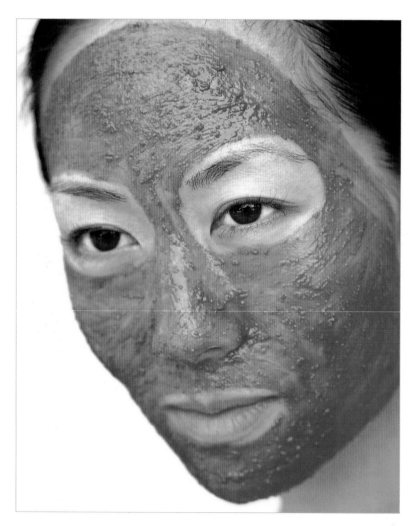

A mixture of honey, avocado oil, and red clay makes a gentle exfoliant.

If you're concerned about acne scarring or sun damage, a relatively new procedure called microdermabrasion offers a more permanent solution. Unlike laser or chemical peels, it's safe for women of color who are prone to hyperpigmentation. The procedure takes about thirty minutes and is offered by dermatologists and beauty professionals. You'll need to book at least six sessions to see lasting results, but there's literally no down time. The technician operates a device that emits a stream of finely shaped crystals that gently polish dull and damaged skin, reducing fine lines, wrinkles, and pore size.

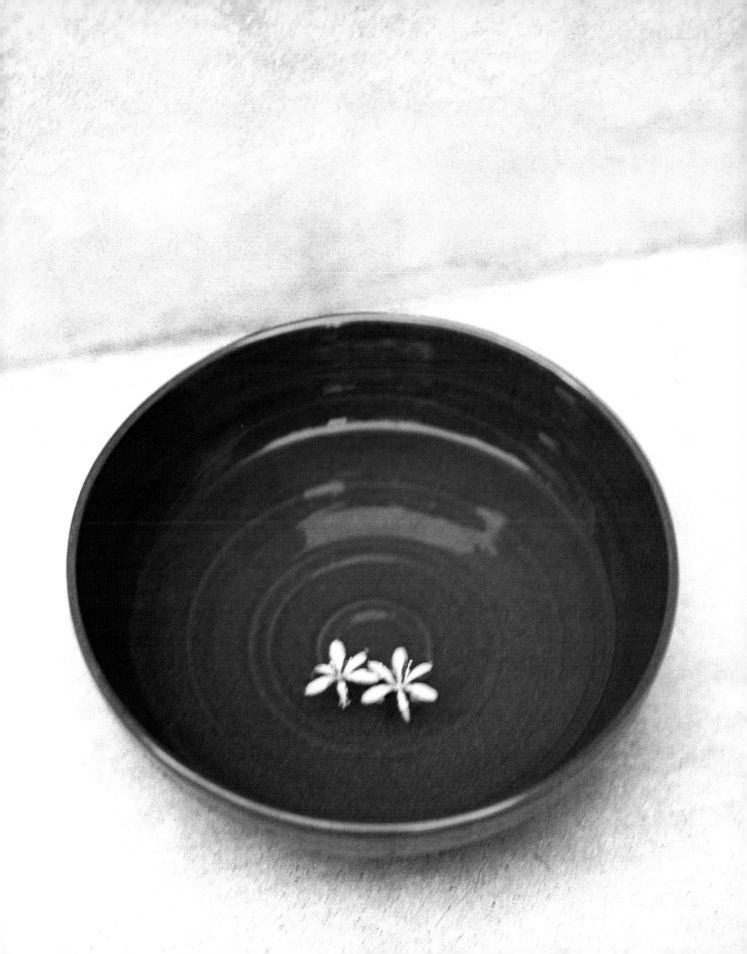

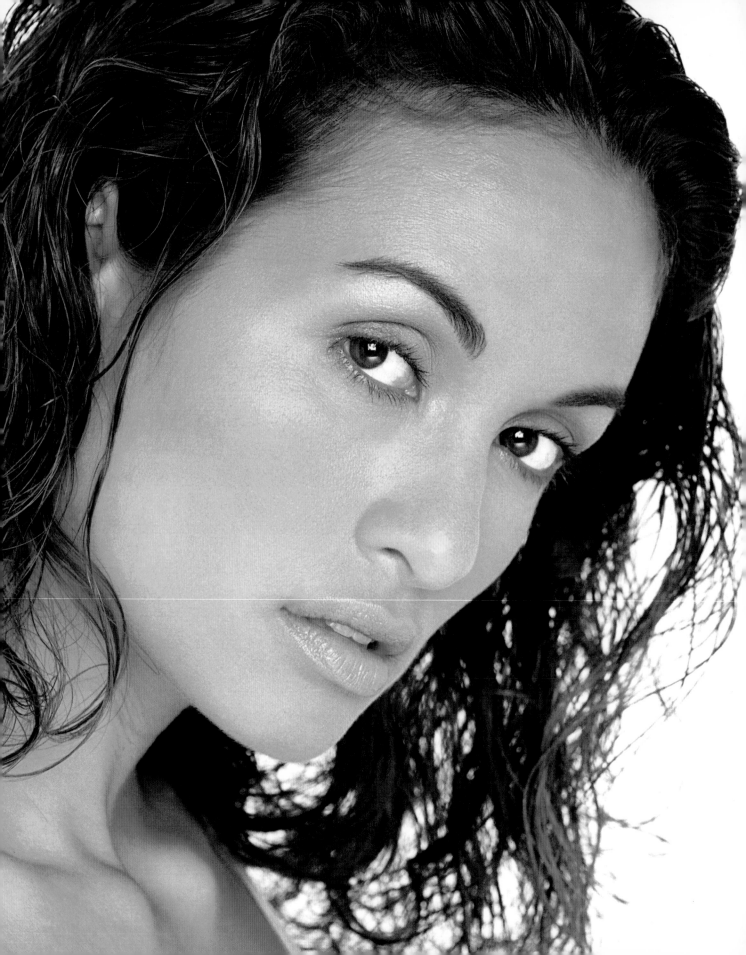

BASIC TRAINING

To keep skin in optimum condition, follow this simple procedure:

MORNING

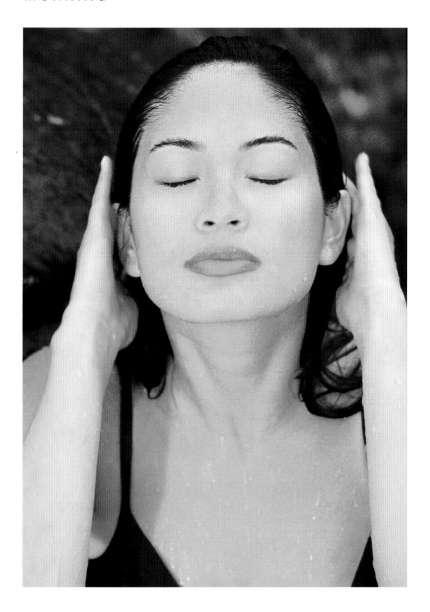

* Wash your face with a gentle cream cleanser.

* You'll get the full benefits of your moisturizer if you apply toner first. It helps the ingredients to penetrate the skin more effectively.

* Always apply a treatment (a serum or ceramide capsule) before applying your moisturizer.

* Apply moisturizer, working it into the throat and neck.

* Use your fingertips to apply eye cream, preferably one with an SPF 10.

NIGHT

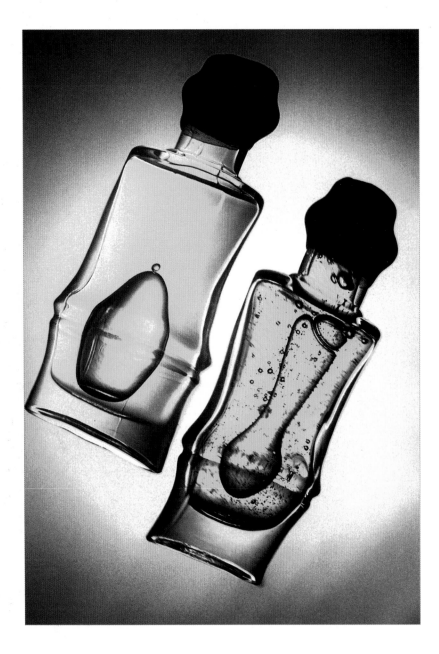

✳ Wash the face.
There's no need to tone again.

✳ Apply a night cream
without an SPF.

✳ Apply an eye cream
without an SPF.

ONCE A WEEK

✳ Use a mask for your skin type.
Unlike exfoliants, which slough
off dead skin cells, masks are
designed to rehydrate dry skin
or soak up excess oil and
tighten pores. Because oily
skin is very rare among Asian
women, Famularé doesn't
recommend using a clay mask.
Instead, choose a cream-
based formula containing algae
or plant extracts. A good time
to apply a mask is while you're
in the bathtub. The heat and
steam will help the ingredients
to penetrate more deeply.

✳ To remove the mask, soak a
washcloth in tepid water and
press it down on the face.
Avoid dragging the washcloth
over your skin.

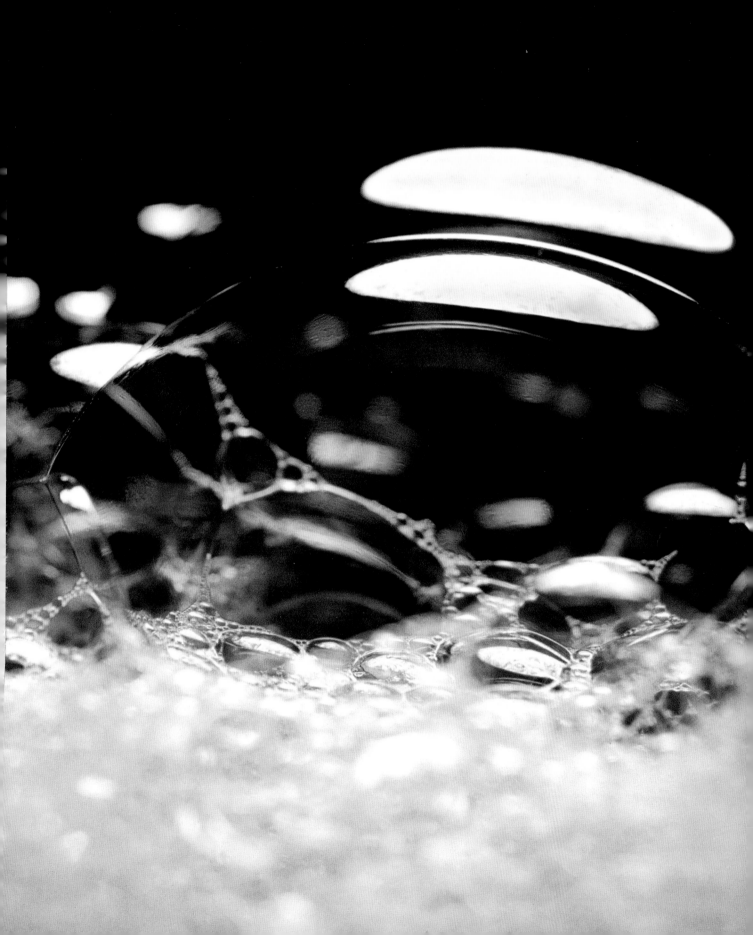

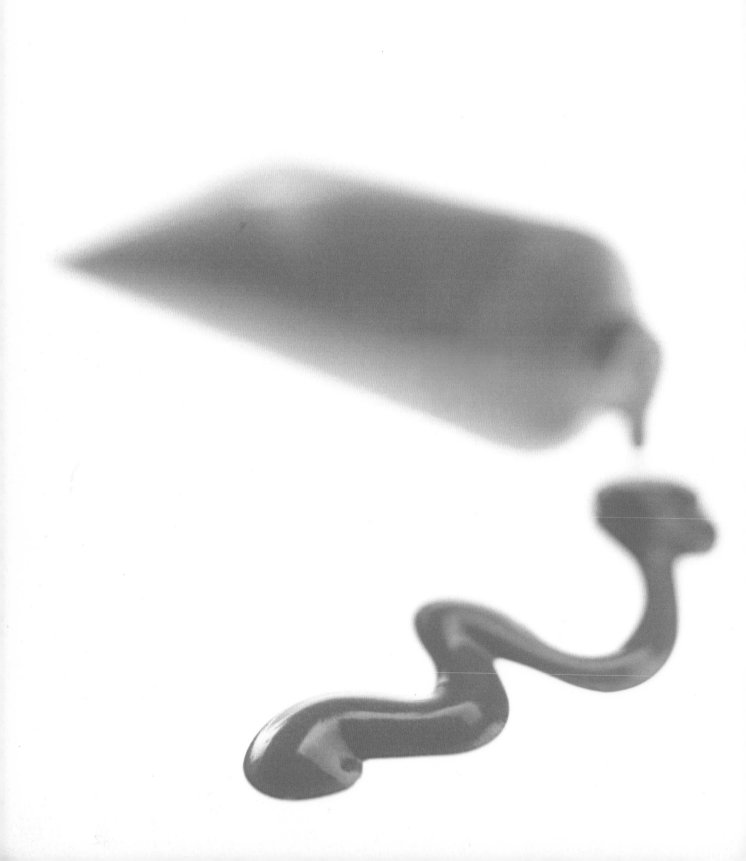

FIRST, BASE 4

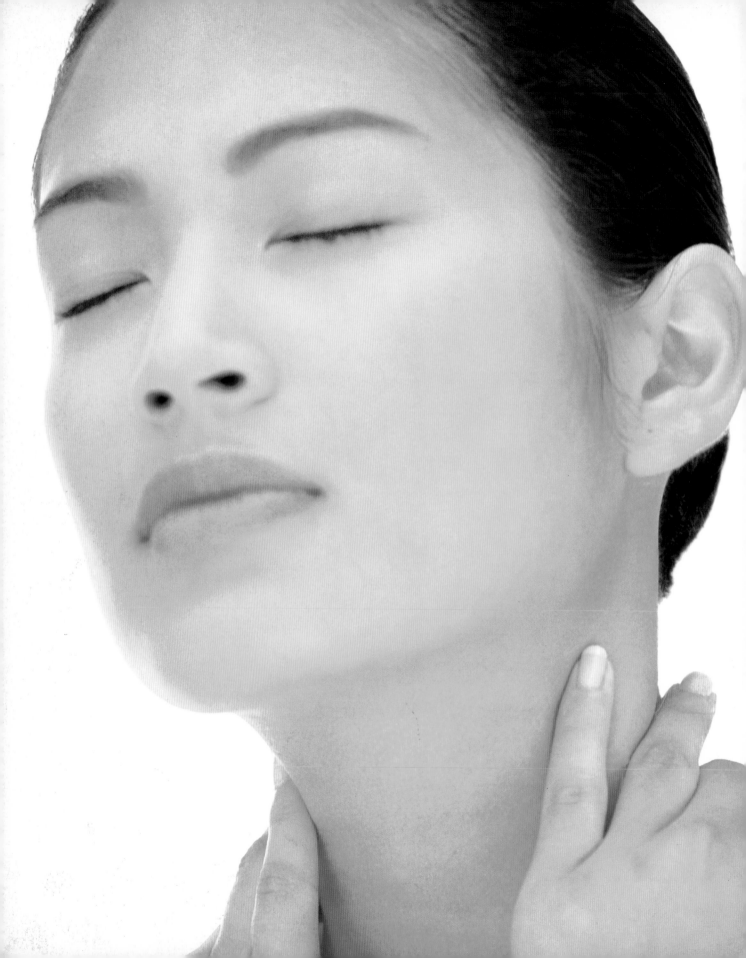

THERE ARE SO MANY LOOKS YOU CAN
ACHIEVE WITH FOUNDATION (ALSO
CALLED BASE), AND THEY TEND TO
GO IN AND OUT OF FASHION EVERY
FEW YEARS. THE MATTE FACE WAS IN
FOR A WHILE, THEN IT WAS ALL ABOUT
TRANSPARENT, SEE-THROUGH SKIN.
NOW MATTE IS MAKING A COMEBACK.
THE IMPORTANT THING TO REMEMBER
IS THAT FOUNDATION WAS CREATED
TO EVEN OUT SKIN TONE AND
CAMOUFLAGE MINOR IMPERFECTIONS.
BUT IT ALSO ACTS AS A PRIMER, CRE-
ATING A NEAR-PERFECT CANVAS UPON
WHICH TO APPLY OTHER COLORS—

Custom blending is one solution for bi racial women like Young, who have trouble finding an over-the-counter foundation that matches their skin tone.

eye shadow, lipstick, blush. If your skin is in pretty good shape and you don't feel that you need foundation, just use a light concealer where necessary and dual-finish powder.

Asian women have always had trouble finding foundations that match their skin tones. That's because most of the products on the market have pink undertones. My rule of thumb: you can never have too much yellow in your foundation. In fact, when I created my own line of products, Margaret Kimura Cosmetics, I made sure that the company offered a wide range of shades to accommodate every possible skin tone.

Before you even think about applying foundation, make sure your skin is clean. After all, you wouldn't paint on a dirty canvas, would you? It's also a good idea to wait a few minutes after moisturizing before you apply your makeup so the foundation "stays put."

If you're not used to wearing foundation, you may worry that you'll look like you're wearing a mask, but the idea is to master the art of application so your skin will actually look better, almost translucent. To me, putting on foundation is like building a house. You're creating a strong structure for the house you're building—that's why they call it foundation.

If your complexion is good, you can get away with a foundation that provides light to medium coverage.

COUNTER INTELLIGENCE

If you're like most women, you might be tempted to throw up your hands in desperation when you visit the makeup counter. Should you choose a liquid or a cream foundation? Oil-free or oil-based? And what the heck is dual-finish foundation anyway?

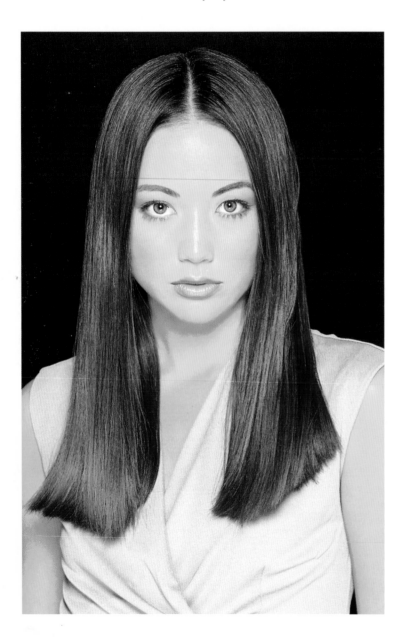

First and foremost, it's important to know your skin type. The most common types are dry, oily, acne-prone, or combination skin, which simply means that you're oily in the T-zone (nose and chin) and drier on the rest of your face. If your skin is acne-prone, it's best to stick with formulations that don't have a lot of excess oils in them. The same goes for combination skin. Still, it's important to moisturize before applying foundation. My advice, unless you have extremly dry skin is to choose an oil-free moisturizer, then follow-up with an oil-free foundation. There are also a few other factors to take into consideration when choosing a foundation. Acid peels or sun damage can create hyperpigmentation—dark spots on the face and neck. Overexposure to the sun can also result in heavy freckling. To camouflage these problems, you'll need a product that provides heavier coverage, like a cream or a dual-finish foundation.

I went through a phase where I'd ask my friends and clients to let me examine their makeup bags. What I discovered was that almost every one of them was using the wrong foundation. Some of them had oily skin, yet they were using an oil-based foundation. Or they were using a product that provided way too much coverage for their skin. So that you won't make the same mistake, I've developed these guidelines to help you make the right choice:

LIQUID: There are two types of liquid foundation: oil-free, intended for oily or acne-prone skin, and oil-based, a good choice for skin that needs a little extra moisture.

CREAM: Available in stick or pancake form. I don't recommend them because they tend to be a lot heavier than other types of foundation, but mature women or those with very dry skin may do well with them if they don't overdo it.

DUAL-FINISH: May be applied wet (for lighter coverage) or dry (for heavier coverage). They're also great for touching up your makeup at the end of the day.

COLOR BALANCERS: Available in green, yellow, and red, they're designed to even out skin tone, but Asian women generally don't need them.

IF YOUR SKIN IS OILY: Choose a water-based formula.

IF YOUR SKIN IS DRY: Choose an oil-based formula.

IF YOU HAVE COMBINATION SKIN: Choose a water-based formula or a dual-finish formula and use it dry on oily areas and wet on the rest of the face.

TO FIND OUT WHAT SHADE YOU NEED: Dab a little foundation on the inside of your wrist. The skin there most closely matches your natural underlying skin tone. My Number One Rule: you can never have enough yellow in your foundation, no matter what your ethnicity. Asian women: avoid pink tones like the plague. You'll look garish.

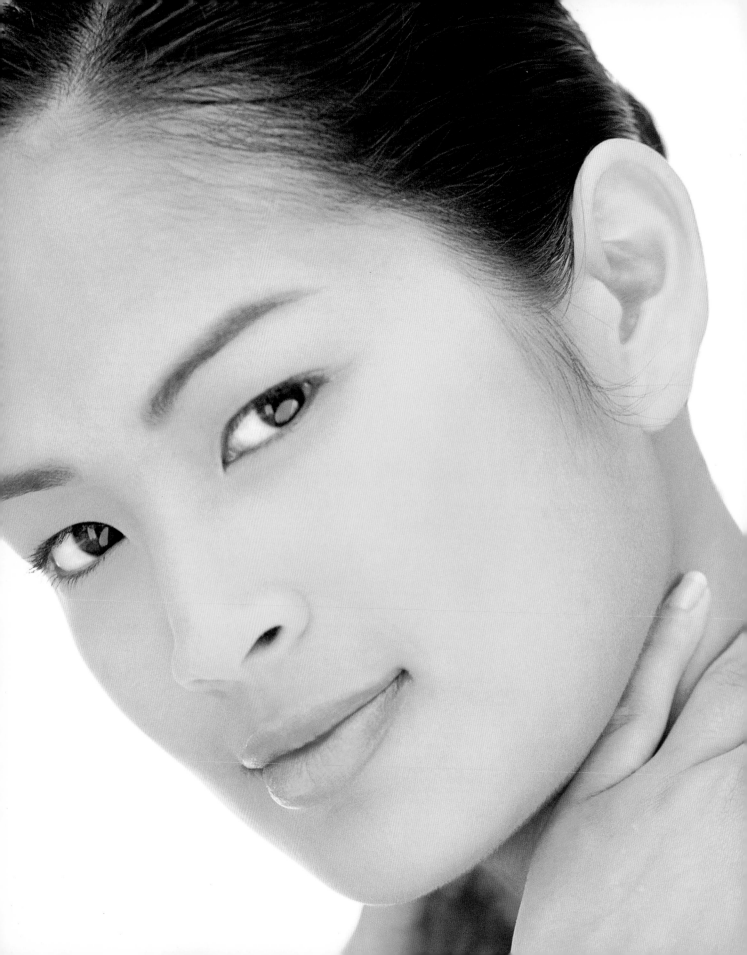

READY, SET, GO

Start by examining your face in the mirror, looking for dark under-eye circles, blemishes, or any discoloration that needs extra coverage. Dab a little concealer on those spots first. While it's perfectly acceptable to apply concealer with your fingers, a brush makes it easier to blend it into hard-to-cover areas.

I prefer using a sponge to apply foundation because it helps prevent too much being applied. I can also cover more area faster and more evenly than I could with my fingers. Another plus: my sponge lets me blend foundation into areas that are hard to get to, like the hairline, underneath the eyes, over the eyelid, and in the crease of the nose or neck—the areas that people typically neglect.

Just remember that most women need two different shades of foundation: a lighter shade for the winter months when they're not getting as much sun and a darker shade for the summer months. My advice is to buy several shades and blend them to adapt to your skin tone as it changes.

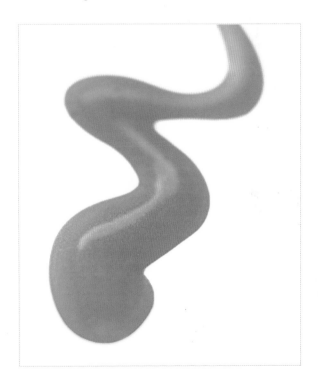

WHY DO YOU NEED FOUNDATION?

1. To balance and even out skin tone. 2. To camouflage minor flaws. 3. As a primer to create a canvas on which to apply other colors.

1

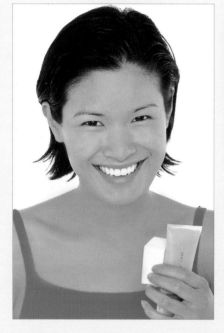

2

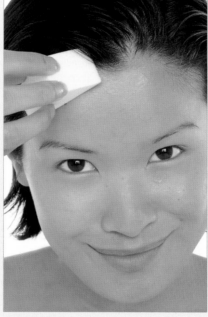

3

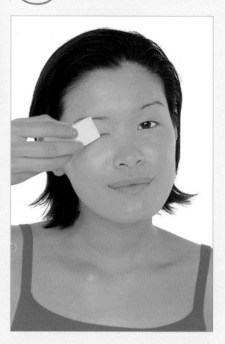

Use a latex sponge to apply foundation. You can pick them up in any drugstore or beauty supply store, and you'll find them invaluable for covering a large area quickly and evenly. Another plus: the triangle-cut latex sponge lets you get into those hard-to-reach areas like under the lash line and around your nose. Because they are so inexpensive, I generally discard them after one or two uses, but you can extend the life of your latex sponges by washing them with a mild soap and water.

Start your application by applying foundation to the forehead. Using the tip of your latex sponge, gradually work the excess foundation into the hairline. This step is even more important if you wear your hair off of your face or will be pulling it back into a ponytail or chignon.

Don't forget the eyelids. Think of it as prepping a wall before you paint. Your eye shadow will not only last a lot longer, the colors you choose will look truer.

4

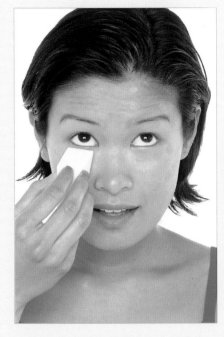

5

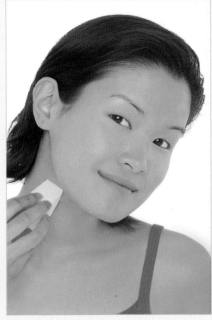

6

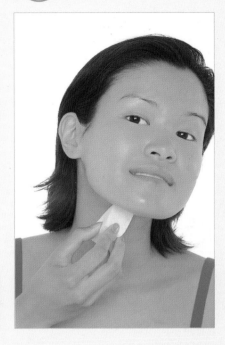

Use your sponge to blend foundation under the lash line, getting as close to the lashes as possible. Again, you're priming the canvas and evening out the skin tone. Since I prefer powders to pencils for lining the eyes, I find that priming the under-eye area with foundation first helps my eyeliner stay put.

Continue to blend the foundation along the neck, which is actually a part of the face. Again, the idea is too even out the skin tone so there's no visible line of demarcation between the face and neck.

Similarly, it's important to blend foundation below the jawline as well. This is one area most women tend to overlook, but if you take your time and complete all six steps, your results will be that much more professional.

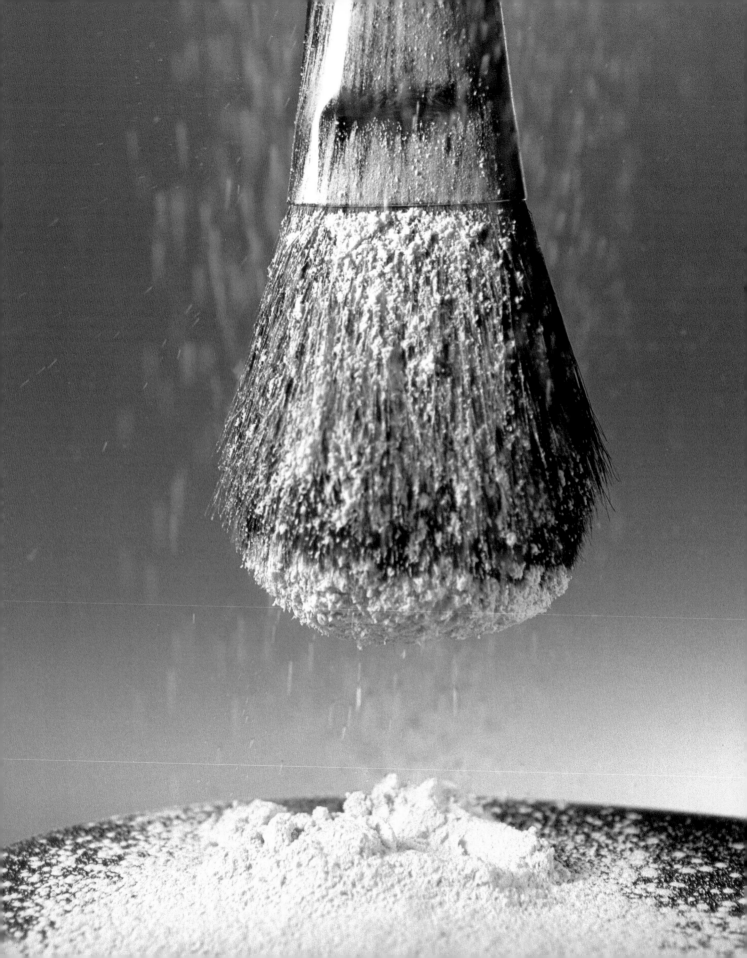

POWDER

Powder has a couple of different uses. First and foremost, it's essential for setting your makeup—it's the very first thing you do after applying foundation. I also use powder to create a softer look when I'm working with an intense, high-pigment cheek color. The trick is to dip your blusher brush into a little loose powder first, then into the color. Finally, by going back over the face with my powder brush after completing the eyes, cheeks, and lips, I can blend all the colors together.

Powder is available in different formulas, each of which is designed for a very specific purpose. Use these guidelines to help you know when to use each one.

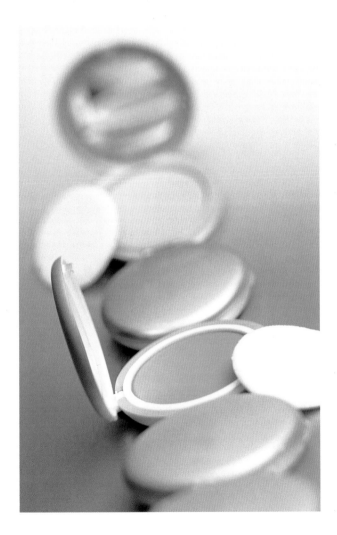

LOOSE POWDER: Designed for heavier coverage. Use your brush to deposit powder onto the face, then use your puff to press or pat the powder into the skin for a flawless finish.

PRESSED POWDER: Usually available in compact form, it's a good touch-up tool to take the shine off your face.

DUAL-FINISH POWDER: Use it wet as foundation or dry to provide heavier coverage.

MATTE POWDER: Use this when you want a flat finish with no hint of shimmer or shine. Not my first choice for very dry skin.

SHIMMER POWDER: Loose powder that adds shimmer or sparkle to the skin. Use a brush, not a puff, to apply. A latex sponge is a great tool for working the powder around the eyes and under the lashes.

WATER POWDER: This is a new category of translucent powder that looks dry but goes on wet to create a dewy complexion.

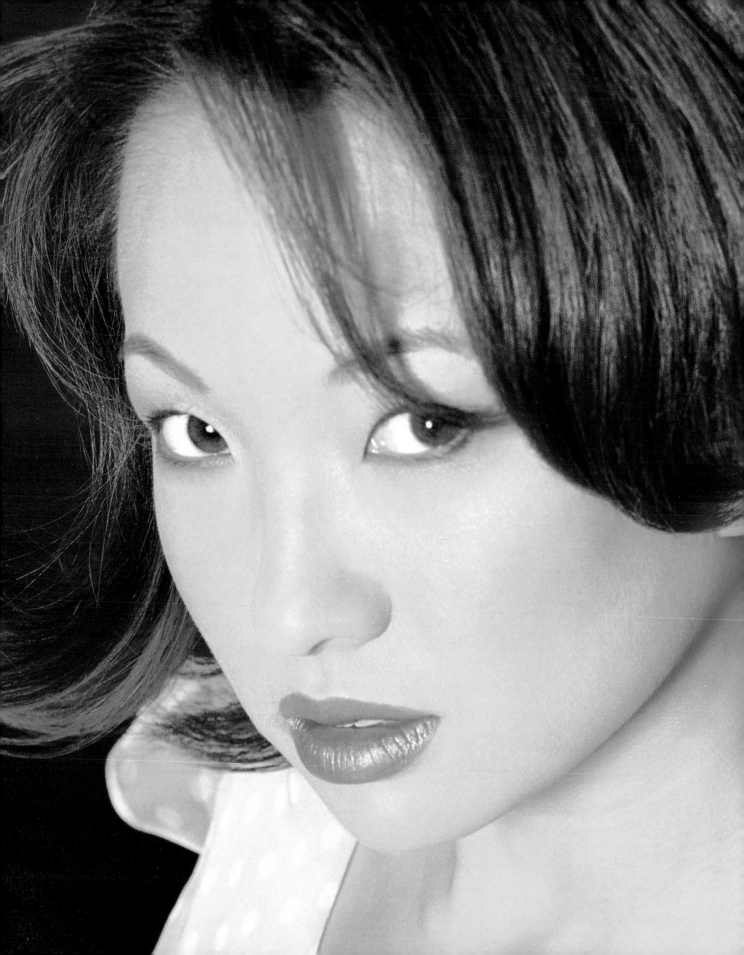

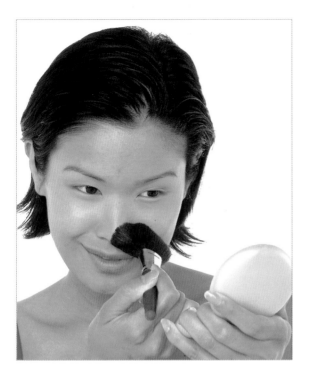

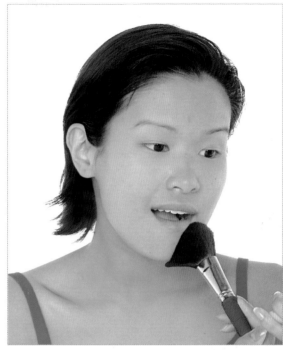

Use a brush to apply the powder evenly over the face.

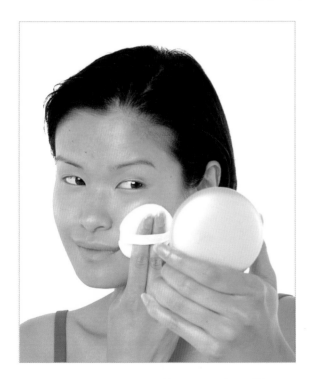

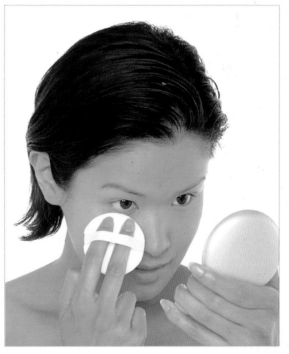

Use a powder puff to press or pat powder into the skin.

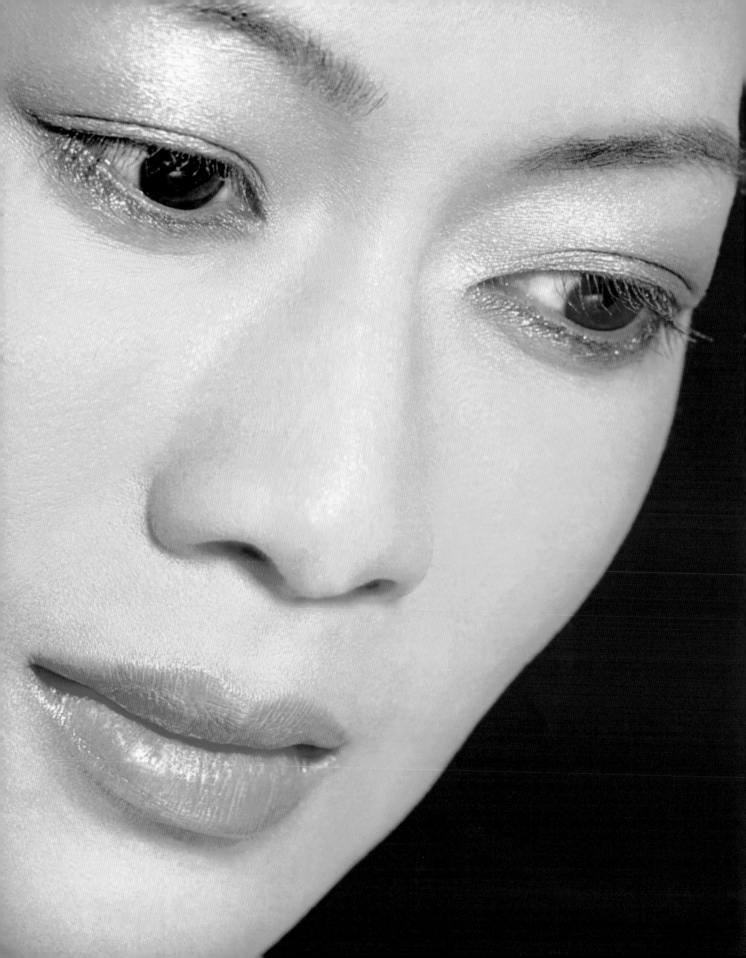

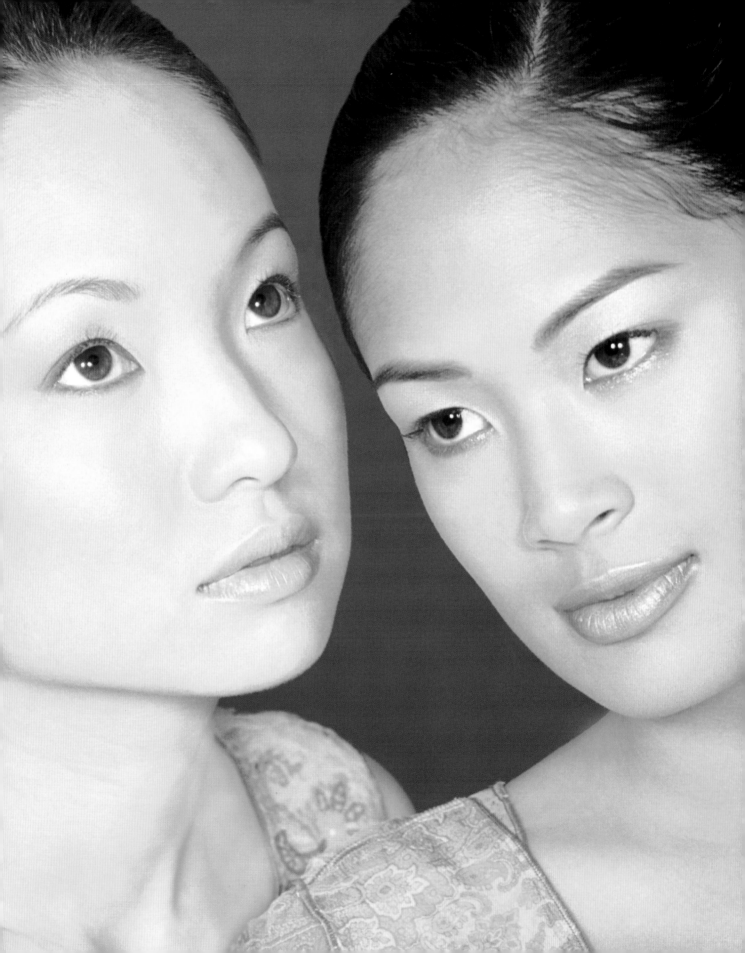

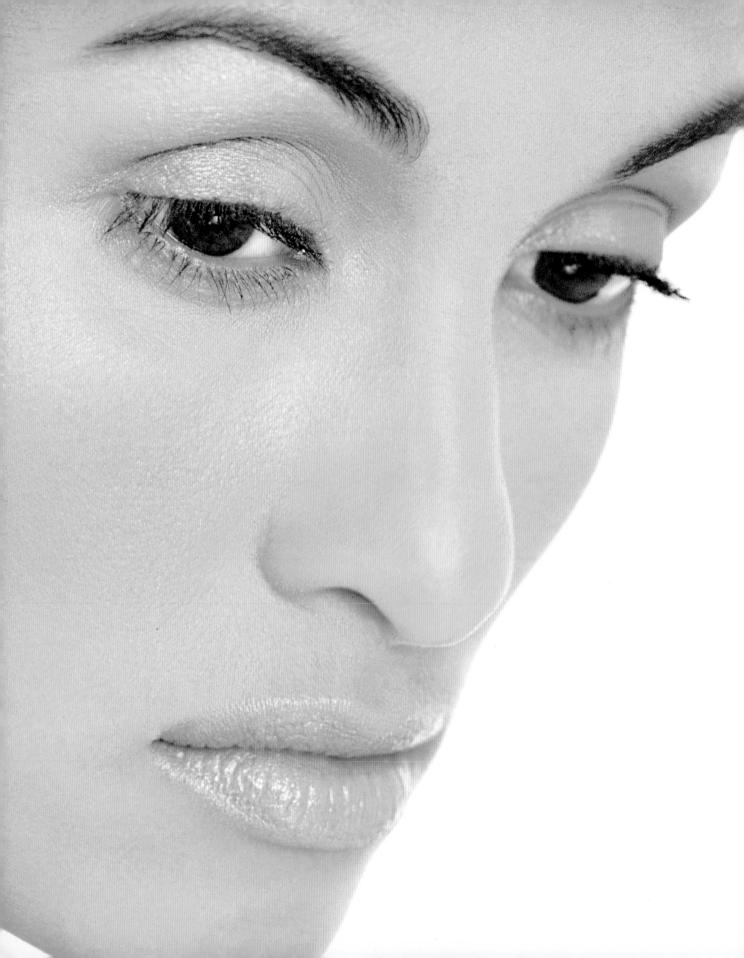

5

IN LIVING COLOR

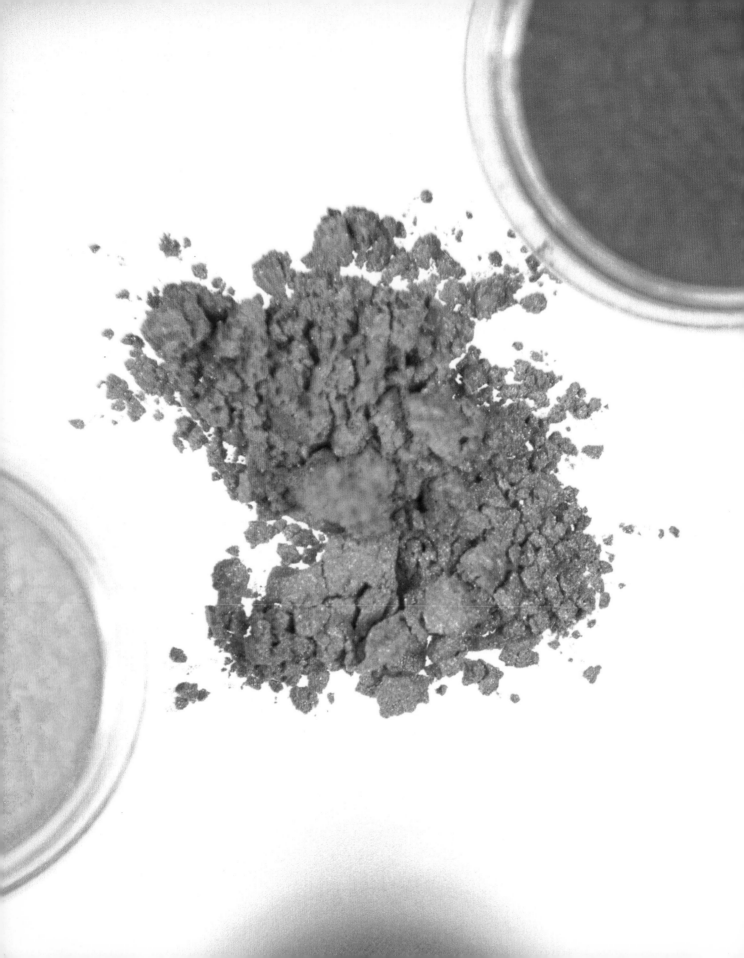

ASIAN WOMEN CAN CARRY OFF BOLD,

DRAMATIC COLOR IN WAYS THAT

OTHER WOMEN CAN'T. THE TROUBLE

IS, NOT MANY OF US ARE BRAVE

ENOUGH TO EXPERIMENT WITH COLOR.

INSTEAD, WE STICK TO THE BASICS—

NEUTRAL SHADES OF BROWN, CREAM,

AND BEIGE. I THINK WHAT SCARES

ASIAN WOMEN ABOUT COLOR

IS THAT THEY DON'T KNOW HOW TO

USE IT. THE POINT IS, IF YOU KNOW A

LITTLE ABOUT TONE, YOU CAN

WEAR ALMOST ANY COLOR YOU WANT.

YOU'RE LIMITED ONLY

BY YOUR OWN IMAGINATION.

Color doesn't have to come on strong. If you're going out to a nightclub, you can be a little more outrageous. But you can also go with pale or pastel shades of blue, green, pink, purple, or even red. If you're using color on your eyes, remember to apply the Shadows and Light technique. You might want to place a highlighted shade of pink on your brow bone and a deeper shade of rose on the outer part of the eyelid.

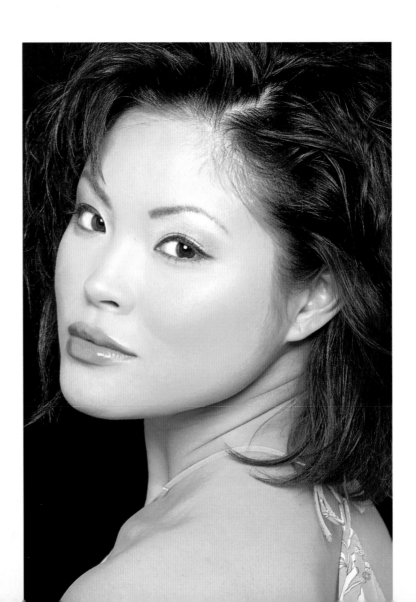

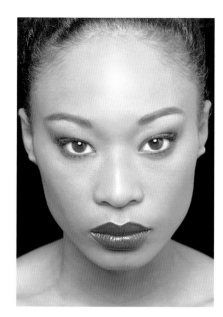

It's also important to balance your eyes and lips. Most Asian women can get by with wearing heavier eye shadow, but the shade of lipstick you choose will determine the intensity of the overall look. Let's say you like dark colors but don't want to wear a nighttime look to the office. The solution is to choose a dark shade of lip gloss instead of a cream or matte lipstick.

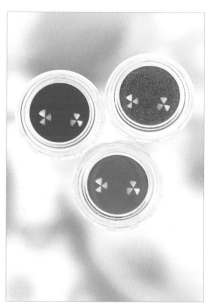

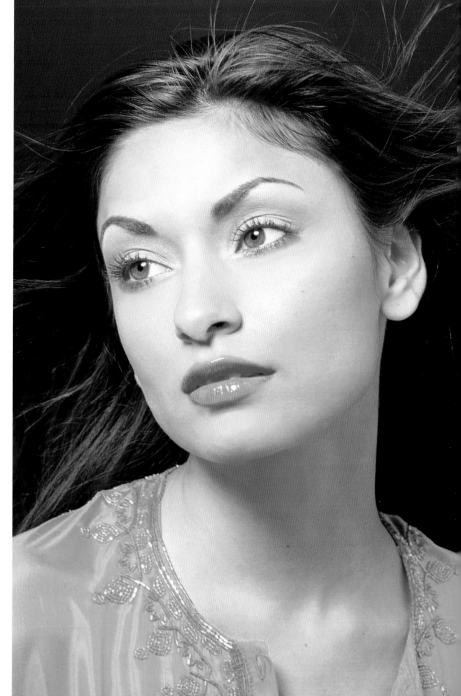

Don't think you can wear green eye shadow? Think again. On occasion it's fun to match your eye shadow to what you're wearing. The idea is to choose soft, shimmery shades.

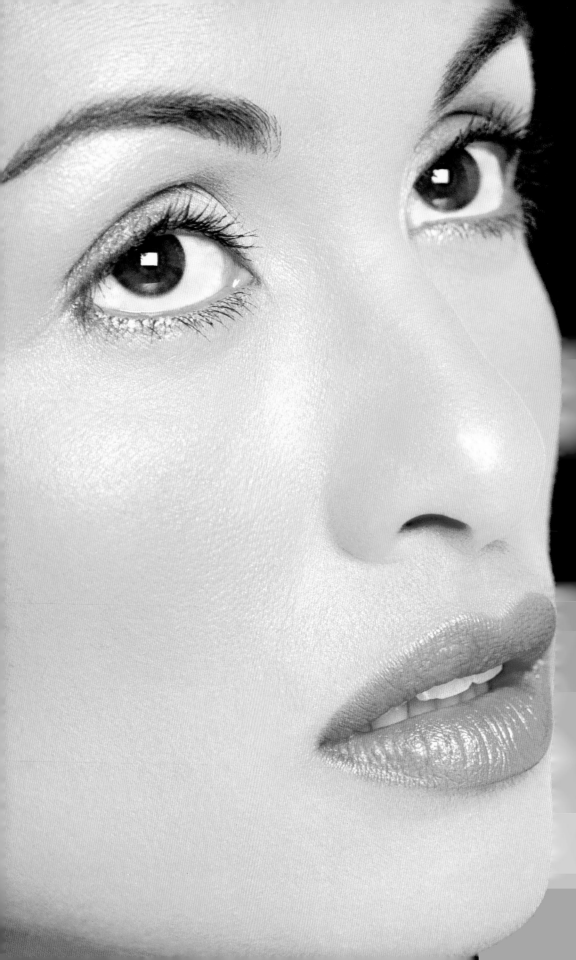

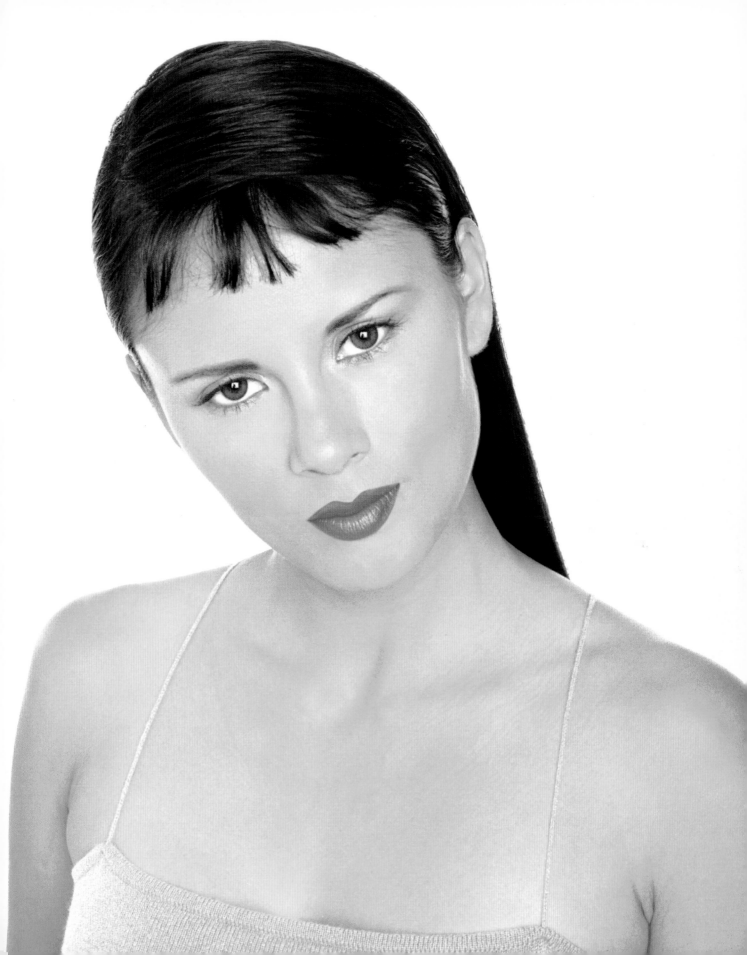

GET CHEEKY

Powder blushes, gels, and bronzers are a great way to add a little color to your cheeks. The problem is that most women tend to be heavy-handed when it comes to blush. Believe me, this is one instance where less definitely is more. My trick is to hit the blusher brush with translucent powder, dip it into the blush, shake the excess off, and apply to the cheek. Remember, you can always add color, so start with just a little.

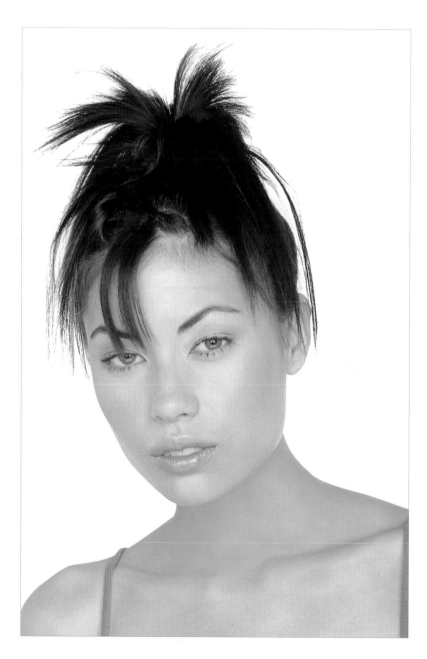

For instance, if you put too much blush on, just dip a latex sponge into a little translucent powder and go over the area to lighten things up a bit. The important thing is to use a light touch when applying blush. Remember, it should never overpower your lip color. The idea is to look like you're blushing, not like you've just been slapped. I have another little trick to balance the eyes and cheeks. I take my eye shadow brush and dip it lightly into my powder blush, then go over the crease of the eyelid just enough to tie the two colors together.

Define and enhance your cheekbones by applying a little highlighter above the cheekbone, then applying blush over it.

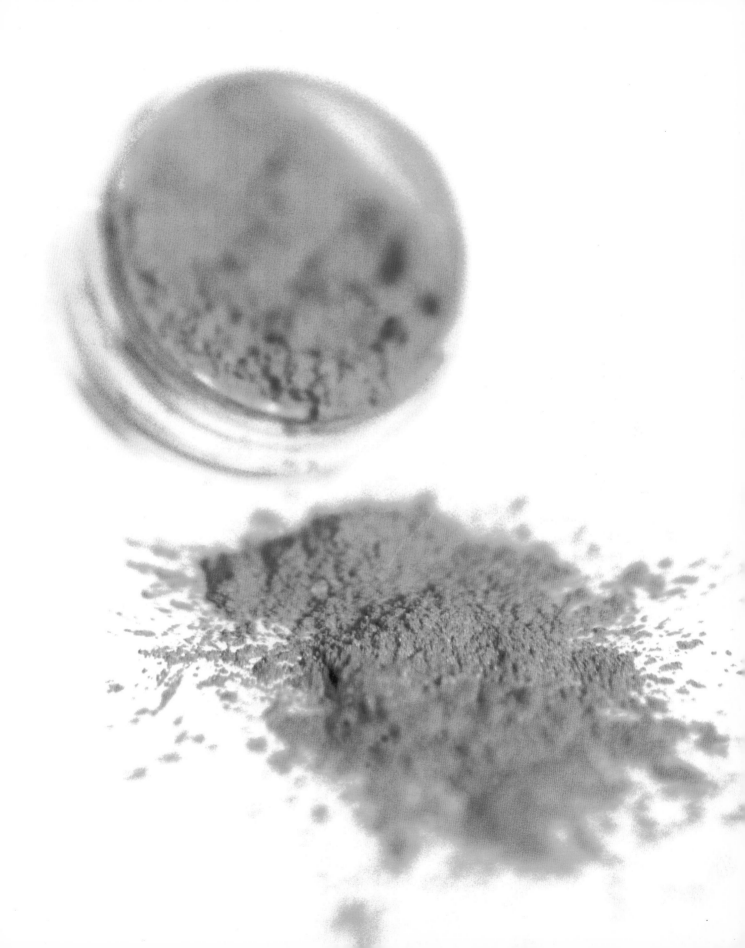

1

2

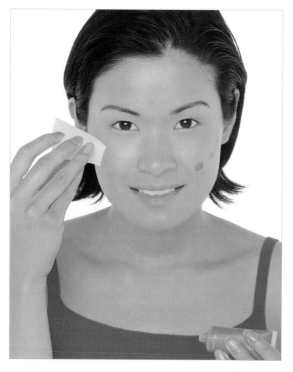

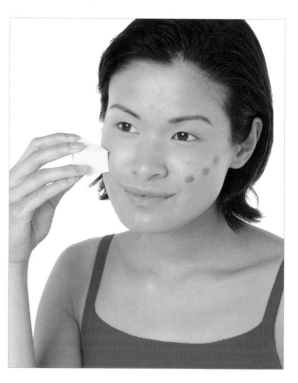

Apply cheek gel with your fingers by dabbing it along the cheekbones.

Use a latex sponge to blend, blend, blend.

Asian women with round faces can define and enhance their cheekbones by applying a little highlighter above the cheekbone, then applying their blush over it. Remember your Shadows and Light technique.

Generally, powder blushes work well to add color to the cheeks, while gel cheek color offers a more transparent look. Still, they can take a little practice since they streak easily. My trick is to mix a little gel cheek color into my foundation and blend it into my cheekbones. If you're not wearing foundation but want a little color on your face, put a dab of cheek gel in the palm of your hand, pat it on the face with a damp latex sponge, and use your thumb to blend it in. The result: a healthy-looking glow that's practically transparent.

One of my favorite new products is a stick-type blush that goes on much as you would apply deodorant. The key is to use a latex sponge to blend the product into the skin once you've applied color where you want it. Other options include powder blush, which works well to add color to the cheeks, and gel cheek color, which offers a more transparent look.

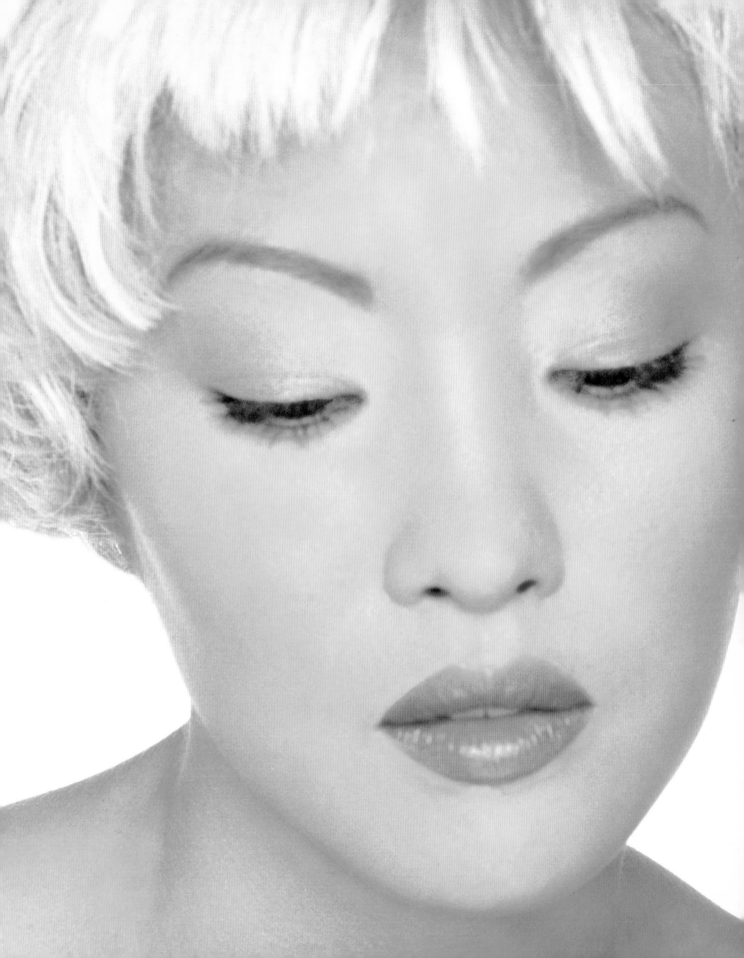

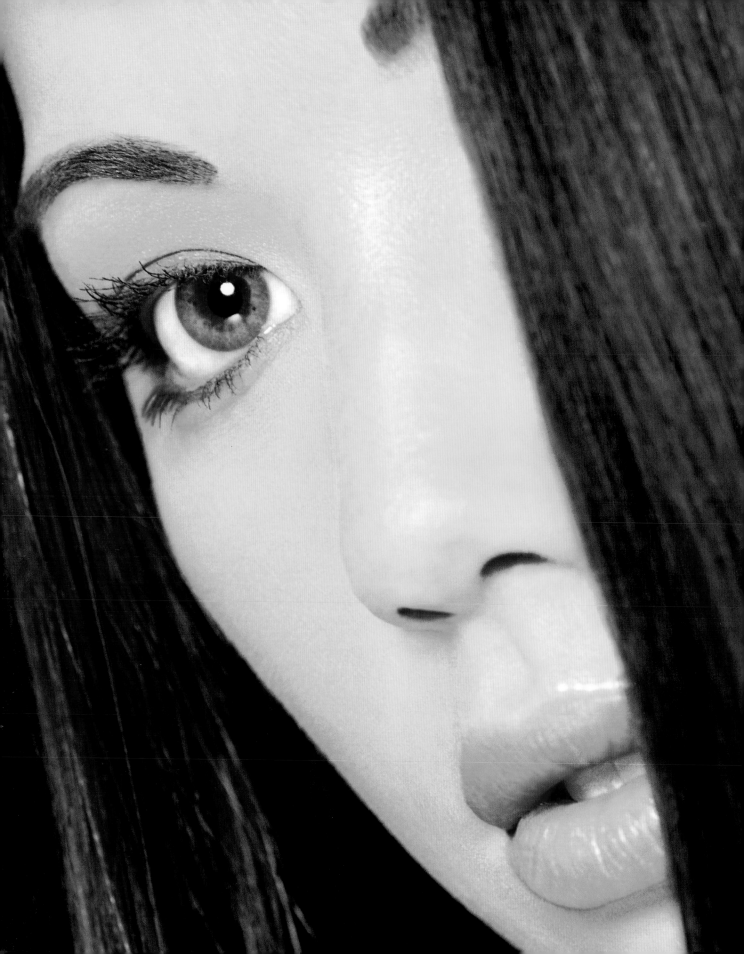

6

THE EYES HAVE IT

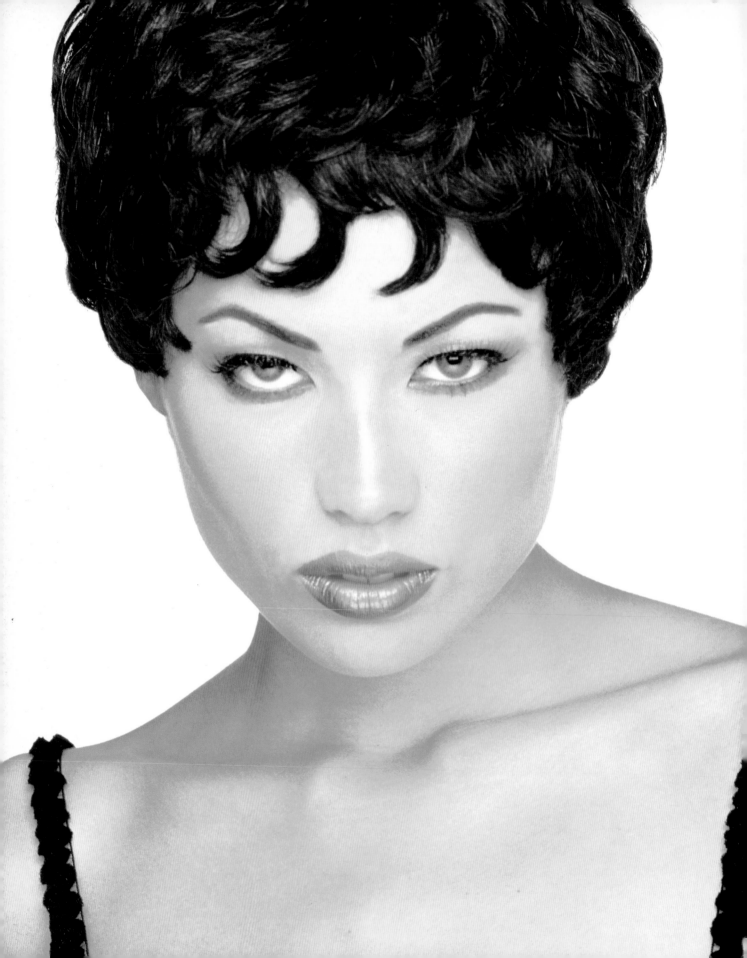

THERE IS SO MUCH ASIAN WOMEN CAN
DO TO PLAY UP THEIR EXOTIC,
ALMOND-SHAPED EYES. WHAT'S
INTERESTING TO ME ABOUT ASIAN
EYES IS THAT WHILE THE CLASSIC
ALMOND SHAPE IS UNIVERSAL, OUR
EYELIDS MAY DIFFER. SOME OF US—
EURASIANS AND AMERASIANS IN
PARTICULAR—HAVE DOUBLE EYELIDS,
WHICH MEANS WE'VE GOT A CREASE.
IF THERE HASN'T BEEN MUCH MIXING
OF CULTURES IN OUR FAMILY, OUR LIDS
MAY HAVE A FLAT SURFACE. LISA LING,
WHO IS PURE-BLOOD CHINESE, COMES
TO MIND. BUT HERS ARE EXACTLY THE

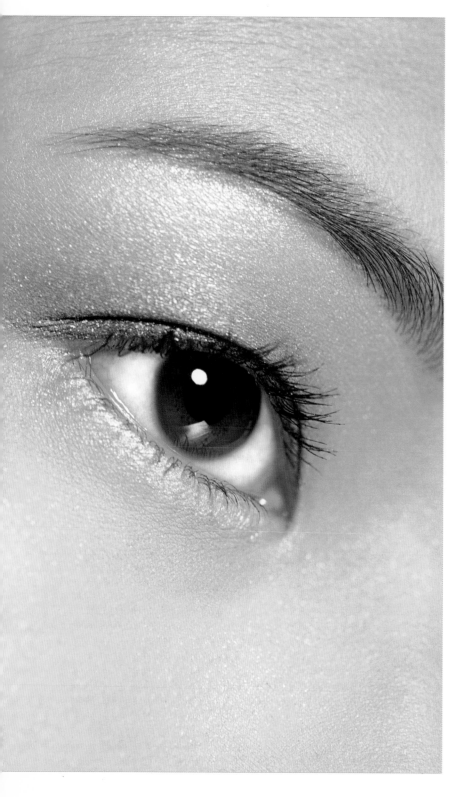

kind of eyes I like to play up using my Shadows and Light technique. By using highlighter on the entire lid, then applying a darker flat tone in the crease, I can create the illusion of a deeper eyelid. Another trick for eyes like these is to use a lighter shade of eyeliner under the lower lashes and a heavier shade to line the lid. The idea is to create more depth on the top lid so the eyes appear to be more open than they really are.

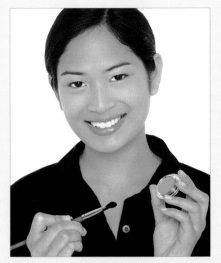

Choose a darker shade of eye shadow and use a full-head shadow brush to apply eye shadow to the bottom part of the eyelid.

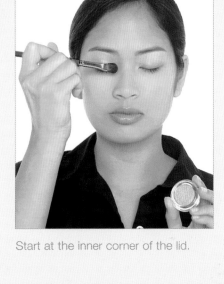

Start at the inner corner of the lid.

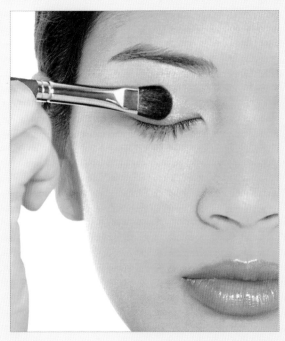

Sweep the brush across the lid.

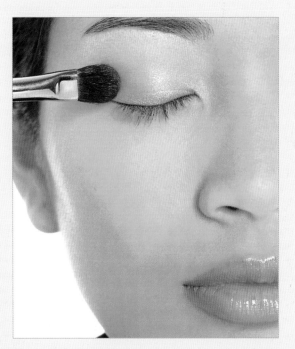

Finish at the outer corner of the eye.

1

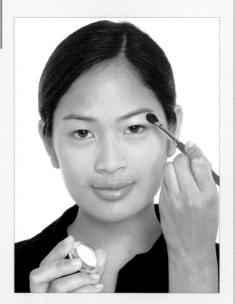

Choose a lighter shade of eye shadow and use a flat-head brush to apply high-lights under the brow bone.

2

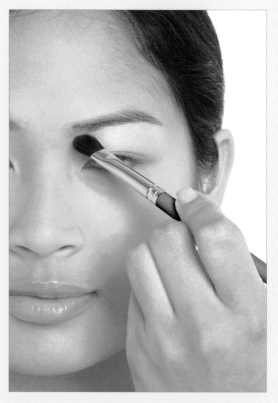

Start at the inner corner of the eye and work your way out.

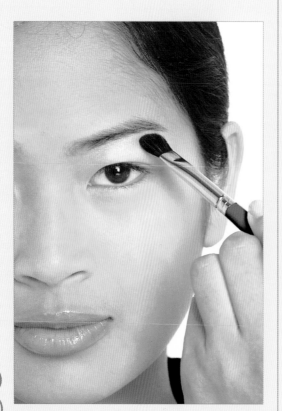

3

Go over your work with the same brush to blend.

My rule of thumb when it comes to eye shadow is to choose a look you're comfortable with, what I call your everyday look, then play around with a couple of other looks. Here are a few you might want to try:

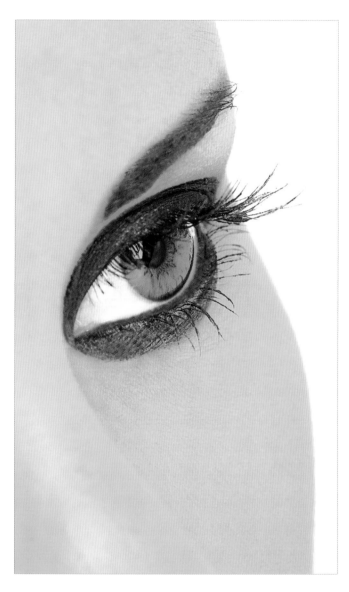

SMOKY EYE: I think smoky eyes are sultry, sexy, and mysterious, but the look isn't limited to shades of black, brown, or gray. You can have smoky burgundies, smoky purples, and smoky silvers. It's the richness of the color, the depth, that lends it that smoky feel. It's a dramatic look, and one that can work at the office if you tone it down a bit. Still, darker shades tend to make features recede, so be careful how dark you go if your eyelids tend to be flat, because really dark shades could make them disappear.

Smoky eyes like this look great on Asian women because they add to our mystery. I use a full-head brush to apply a dark shade of brown or gray eye shadow to the bottom part of the eyelid. The trick is to dampen the brush a little to keep the color from bleeding. After it dries, I go over the area again with a little more shadow. Then I line the lower lid with a wet liner brush and charcoal shadow, wait until it dries, and go over the area again with a flat-head brush and some more shadow, making sure to smudge the line a bit. I use a pearl highlighter on the brow bone. My crease brush lets me blend an ivory shade of shadow in the crease to tie the light and dark shades together. To really blend the colors, I hit my crease brush with a little bit of earth-tone blush and smudge it in the crease.

NATURAL: I think of natural shades as colors that mirror flesh tones, like peach or coral. These shades also tend to be flat, which can make features recede. If you mix one of them with a shimmer highlight powder, you can still look natural but create the illusion that your eyes are bigger than they are. Dab a little highlighter on the brow and on the inner corner of the lid to make it appear that you have more eyelid.

YOU CAN WEAR
THE SAME EYE
MAKEUP
BUT CHANGE
THE ENTIRE
MOOD SIMPLY
BY CHANGING
THE COLOR OF
YOUR LIPSTICK.

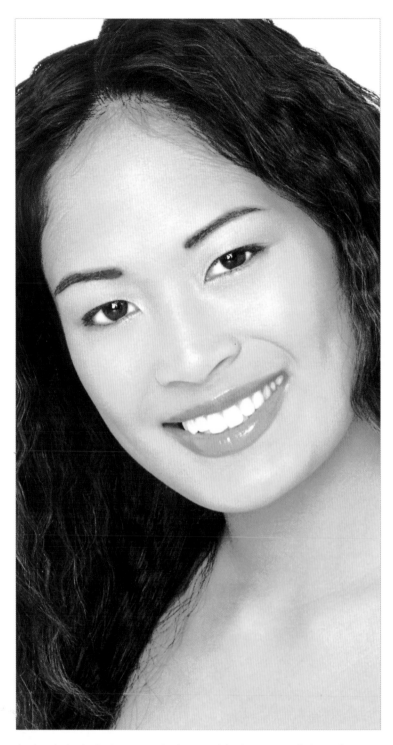

A classic look that can work day or night because all the colors are fresh and neutral.

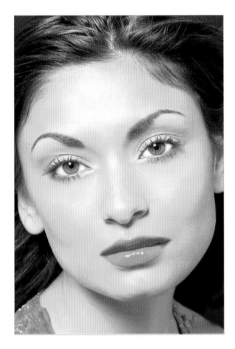

This is a classic daytime/professional look that uses a little more color to make its point. Note the soft metallic green on the eyelid, pearl on the brow bone, and a nutmeg color in the crease for added depth and dimension.

DAYTIME/PROFESSIONAL: This is a no-nonsense, "I mean business" kind of look. It's not sexy or smoky, and it's different from natural, which is almost a see-through look. I think of it as a lighter version of a nighttime look. In fact, you could take this look right from the office to a night on the town by darkening up your eye shadow before you go out. My advice is to wear a lighter shade of your favorite color to the office and wear a deeper shade at night. Remember your Shadows and Light technique when working with darker colors to add depth or drama.

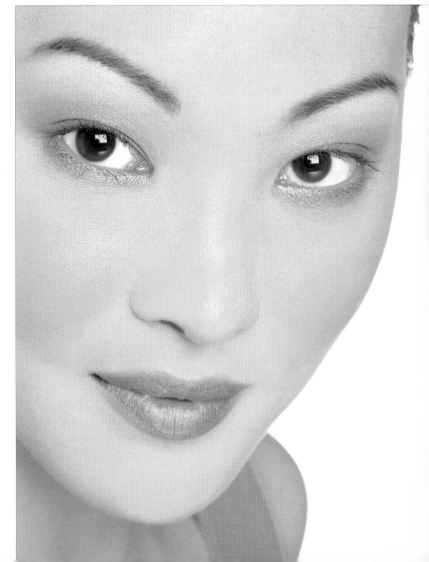

I think of this as an executive look. It's perfectly acceptable for the office, but it's also fun and approachable. I like to use shimmery eye shadow to add a little kick, kind of like wearing the right accessories. Here I used metallic shades of brown and gold on her eyes and an earthy shade of nutmeg in the crease to blend the two shades together. Smudging the shadow just a bit around the eyes creates a softer effect than using eyeliner.

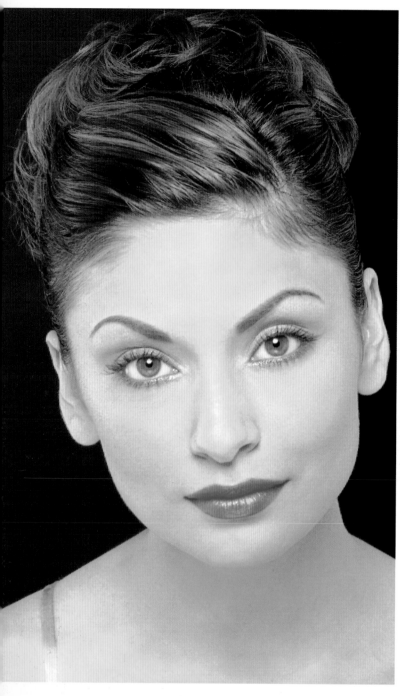

This is a great special occasion look, perfect for a wedding or a gala. With pale shades of lilac and pink on the lids and an opalescent highlighter on the brow bone, the look is soft and feminine. FACING PAGE: For eyes that positively smolder, try using pure pigment mixed with a metallic shimmer.

NIGHTTIME: Depending on what kind of mood you're in, nighttime can mean many things. A girl who's comfortable in natural makeup will still lean toward that look at night. She'll never put false eyelashes on. She'll never wear liquid eyeliner. But she might wear lip gloss with a little shimmer powder or glitter in it. If you love smoky eyes, you would use pencil instead of powder to line the eyes for night—it's much more intense. For a little extra kick, try adding a couple of individual false eyelashes at the outer edge of the eye.

IF YOU WEAR SMOKY EYE MAKEUP DURING THE DAY, WEAR A NUDE LIP SHADE. BUT TO GO OUT AT NIGHT AND CREATE MORE DRAMA, SWITCH TO A DARKER SHADE OF LIPSTICK AND PUT A LITTLE LIP GLOSS ON TOP.

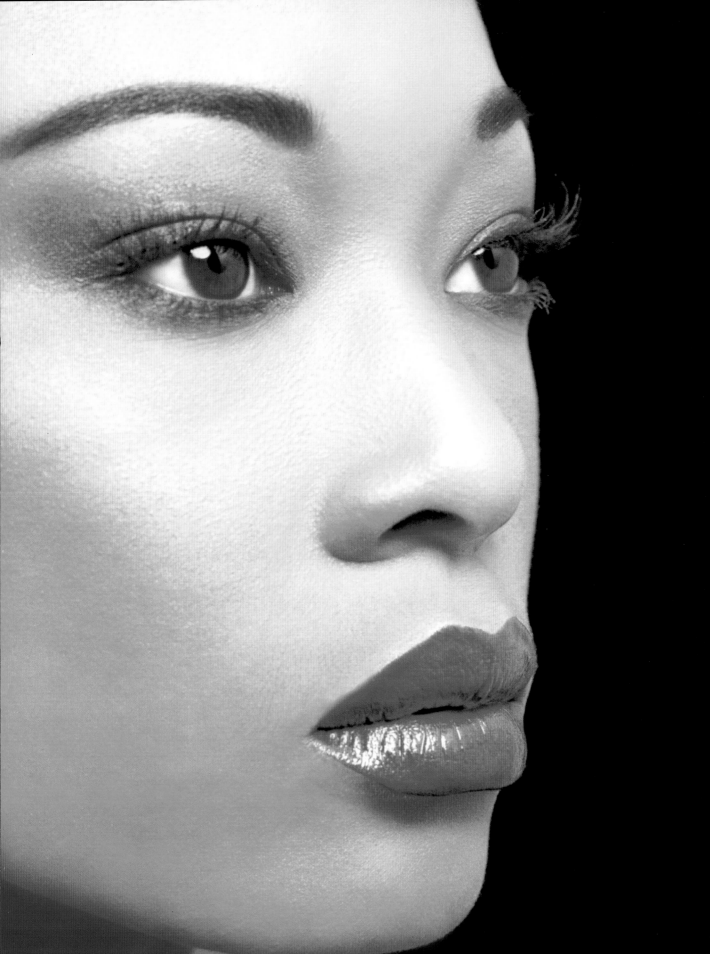

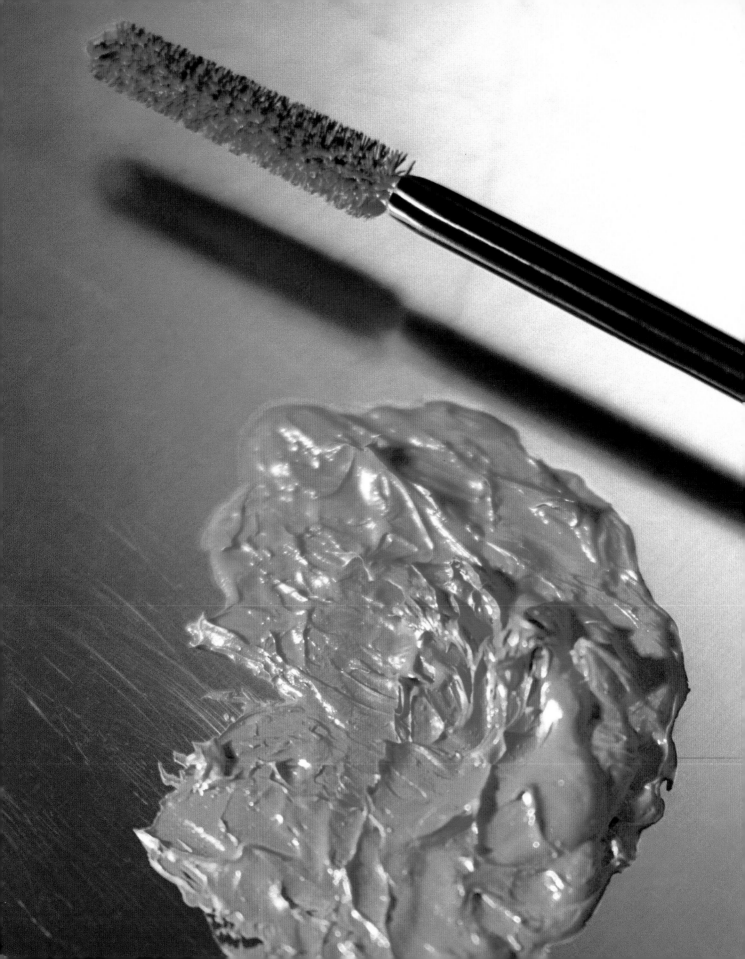

GREAT LASHES

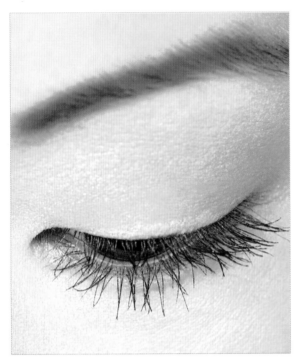

Individual eyelashes open up the eyes and extend the length of your natural lashes.

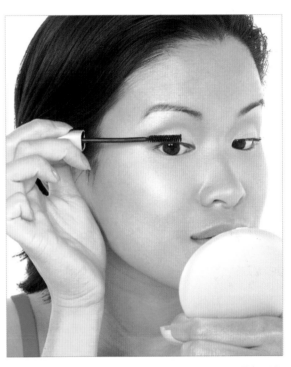

Thinner-tipped wands are best for Asian eyes. They hit the lashes, not the lids, so you'll avoid smudges.

Even if you weren't born with long, lush lashes, they're one of the easiest things to fake. Mascara lengthens and separates the lashes, but more important, it finishes your look. Your eyes will look positively naked if you forget to apply mascara. The most popular shades are black and brown, but if you want to make a statement, choose a vibrant shade of purple or cobalt blue.

Another trick is to apply a few individual eyelashes at the outer corners of the eyes. Many women are afraid to use individual eyelashes since they look so difficult to apply. The fact is, once you get the hang of it, it's amazing how many ways you'll find to use them to improve and enhance your overall look. Applying lashes requires a good pair of tweezers, eyelash glue, and a steady hand. Grab an individual lash with your tweezers, dip the lash into a little eyelash glue, and position the lash where you want it. Hold it there for a few seconds until the glue starts to set.

Individual lashes come in three different lengths: short, medium, and long. For a natural look, choose short- or medium-length lashes. For a more dramatic look, extend the length at the outer edge of the eye with a few longer lashes.

EYE OPENERS

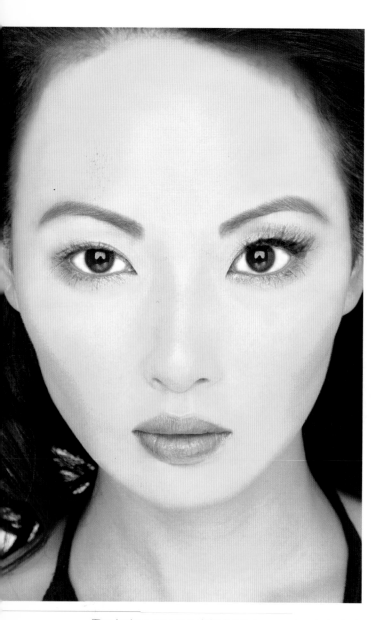

The lashes on your right have been extended. Just look at the difference.

For foolproof results every time, follow this advice:

✳ Apply lashes after foundation, brows, and eye shadow.

✳ Use black eyelash glue so no one will notice where you've attached the individual lashes.

✳ A good pair of tweezers is essential for placing each lash exactly where you want it.

✳ Avoid strip lashes. They look fake and unnatural.

✳ Always curl your natural lashes first so they'll match the curl pattern of the false lashes.

✳ Before affixing individual lashes, apply a light coat of black or dark brown mascara to your natural lashes.

✳ Make sure the individual lashes lean out in the direction of the outer corner of the lash line. It's easier to start the application from the outer corner of the top lash line.

✳ Use wet eyeliner to blend your natural lashes and the false eyelashes together, but make sure the glue has dried before applying eyeliner. Otherwise, you're asking for eyelash disaster.

EYELASH CURLERS

No bag of makeup tricks is complete without an eyelash curler. You will be surprised at how much bigger your eyes look when you curl your lashes first. I have a trick for getting the curl to hold when using a standard pair of metal eyelash curlers. Use your blow dryer to heat the metal head. It has the same effect as putting hot rollers in your hair. But be careful that the metal doesn't get too hot, or you could burn your eyelid.

An even better solution for Asian women is the new heated eyelash curlers. Since our lashes tend to be very straight and thick, they tend to resist taking a curl. The heat generated by these new appliances creates a beautiful bend that stays put all day and night.

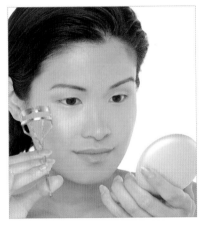
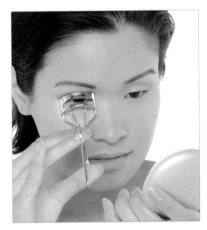
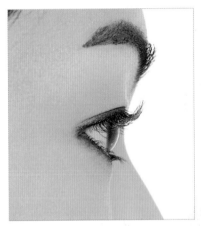

Curling lashes is essential for Asian women because it opens up our eyes. To use a standard metal eyelash curler, open the jaws of the curler, insert it over your lashes, press lightly, and hold for about ten seconds. Be careful not to pull your own lashes out when removing the eyelash curler.

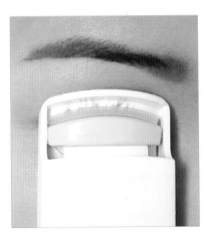
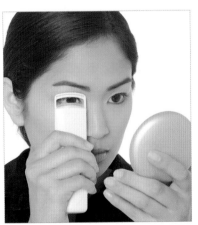
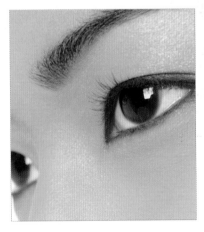

I love the new heated eyelash curlers. They're battery-operated and work like a curling iron. Not only does the curl stay in all day, the heat makes it easier to curl Asian lashes, which tend to be straight and coarse.

DRAWING THE LINE

I love eyeliner because it makes Asian eyes look even more mysterious. Since my style tends to be soft and approachable, I prefer to use powder to line the eyes. But there are several options, and you may prefer something else.

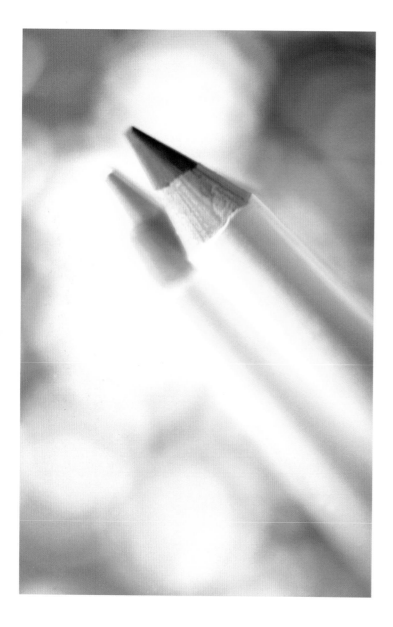

POWDER: A very soft, natural look, plus powders are easy to blend. A great brush is key.

PENCILS: A somewhat stronger look than you'd get with a powder, and it's essential to have a good sponge-tipped applicator or brush to smudge the line after you're done.

LIQUID: Great for nighttime, but it's unforgiving. You've got to have a very steady hand because it's almost impossible to correct mistakes. Liquid eyeliner comes in a bottle with its own brush, but you can also use powdered eye shadow wet to get a similar effect. If so, make sure to invest in a great brush. Look for soft yet firm bristles and a precise cut or edge to keep liner close to the lashes.

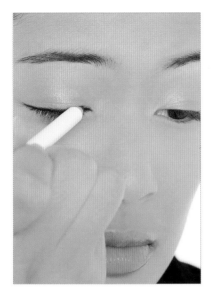

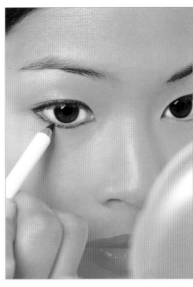

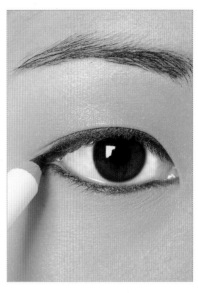

To apply pencil eyeliner start at the inner corner of the eye.

Line underneath the lower lashes in the same way.

Continue to the outer corner so the two lines meet.

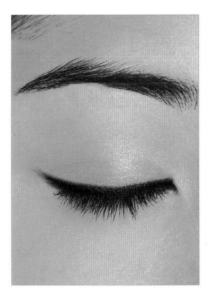

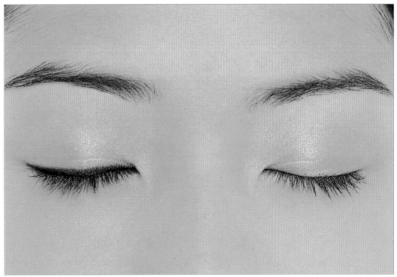

The line should be close to the lashes.

See the difference now that I've lined her right eye.

GIRLS WHO WEAR GLASSES

If you wear heavy frames, you can wear heavier eye makeup and not feel like you're wearing too much. If you wear wire frames or rimless frames, you can be more daring with color. If you're farsighted, get a good magnifying mirror to do your eye makeup. Make sure you blend well, especially if your prescription is strong and will magnify your results.

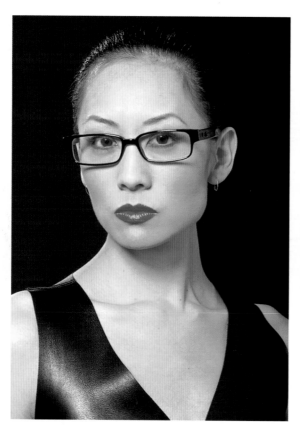
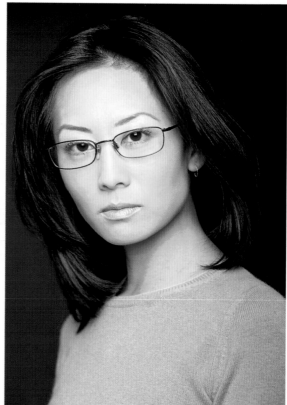

BROWS

Like hairstyles, brow shapes go in and out of fashion. In the 1930s, when "thin was in," women literally shaved off their own brows and painted new ones in. Then in the 1980s actress Brooke Shields created a stir by letting her thick brows grow wild, and before long every woman in America was copying the look. The trouble with trends is that they tend to range from the sublime to the ridiculous. My advice is not to follow the whims of fashion but rather to enhance the shape of the brows you were born with.

Eyebrows should lend balance to the face, and contrary to popular opinion, one size does not fit all. For example, if you have thick eyebrows but they look in proportion with the rest of your features, I'd clean up the brow line but I'd never alter the basic shape. The goal is to make your eyebrows look natural, only better.

You'd be surprised how easy it is to manipulate the shape of Asian brows if you know how to use powders and soft pencils to fill in sparse areas or elongate brows that are too short or have been overtweezed. My own brows would disappear if I didn't fill them in. I overtweezed for years, and they simply haven't grown back. Still, I'm a big advocate of tweezing, which can work miracles for Asian women. Brows that are unruly or coarse, for example, drag down your features and make you look tired. Plus tweezing can take years off your age. My Japanese clients are usually horrified when I take my tweezers out because they don't tweeze in Japan, they use straight razors to shave their brows. They can't stand it when I start plucking, but I'm committed.

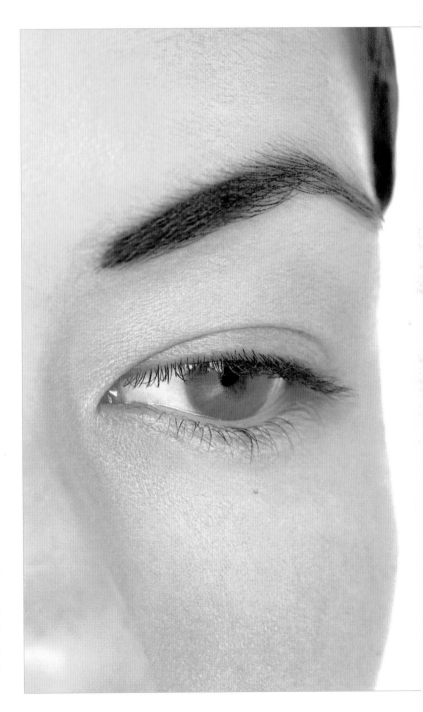

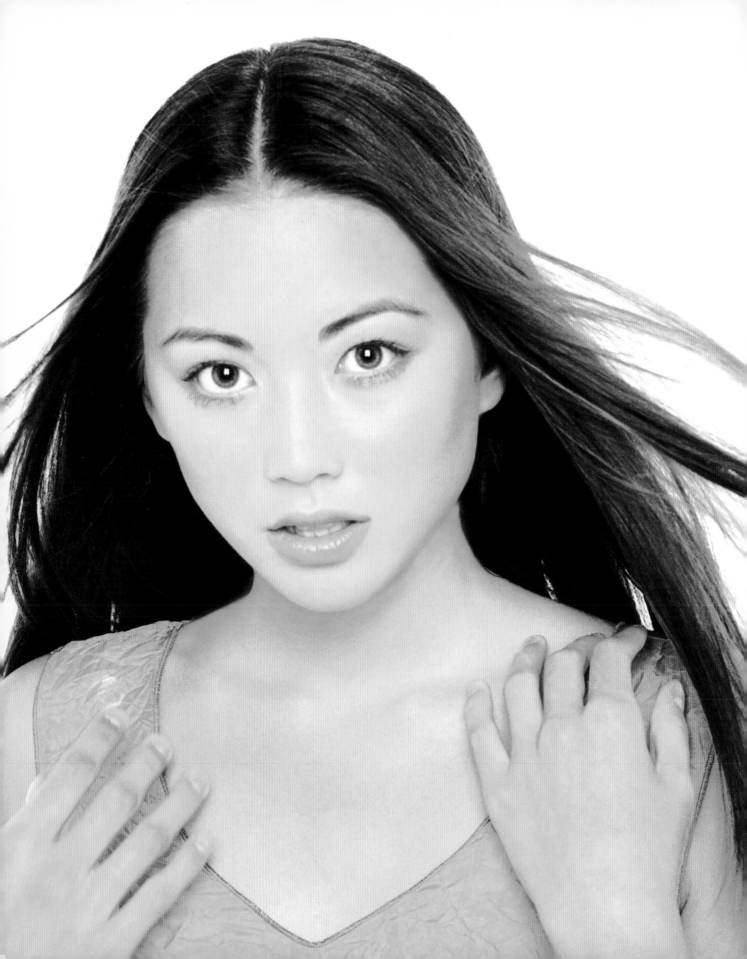

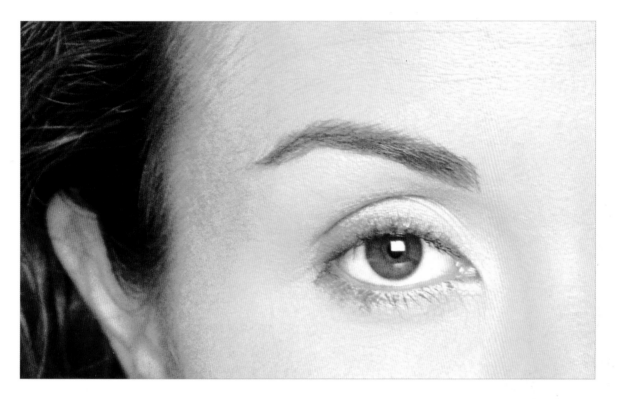

When brows are as great as hers, all that's required is to clean up the strays underneath the brow line to strengthen the shape.

WHY SEE A PRO?

If your brows need a lot of work, I'd suggest making an appointment with a professional—an esthetician or makeup artist—rather than trying to do them yourself. It's a lot easier to maintain your brows at home—tweezing stray hairs below the brow line or between the eyes—once you've got a pattern to follow. Besides, a pro has more experience than you do. She can step back and see the big picture. The goal is to have brows that are in proportion to one another and to the rest of your face. Believe me, it's easy to end up with brows that don't look anything alike once you start whittling away at them.

When choosing a salon, however, make sure it's clean and staffed with professional-looking people. It helps to take along a photo of an actress or model whose brows you admire. Just be realistic. Generally, you can't get the super-duper arch with Asian brows that you can with Caucasian brows. And Japanese, Chinese, and Korean women tend to have unruly brows that don't lie flat and don't arch well either.

WAXING VERSUS TWEEZING

The two most common methods of hair removal are waxing and tweezing. While wax creates a cleaner surface, it's also less forgiving, which is why some estheticians don't use it. Others prefer to wax first in order to remove most of the hair, then go in with tweezers to pick up anything the wax couldn't remove. Because Asian brows are so dark, they can create a blue shadow on the eye area as they grow back, particularly if you have a lot of baby hairs. Waxing can help because it gets all of the hair out at once. Whatever method you choose, you'll need to repeat the process every four to six weeks.

Before applying the wax to your eye area, your esthetician should test the wax to make sure it's not too hot. Blowing on it is not only unprofessional, it's unsanitary. Finally, waxing is not recommended for anyone using Retin-A or Renova, both of which make the skin more sensitive. Be sure to tell your esthetician if you are using either of these medications.

JUST TWEEZING

Invest in a good pair of tweezers so you can maintain your brows between visits to the salon. Asian eyebrows tend to be thick and hard to remove so I'd suggest flat-head tweezers, which can really get a grip on those coarse hairs. Beginners may find that angle-tipped tweezers are easier to manipulate. Here's what you'll need to get started: Sea Breeze or alcohol, an eyebrow brush, aloe vera gel, and your tweezers.

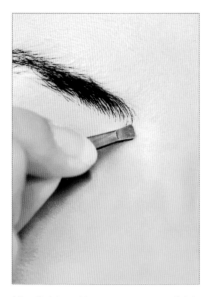

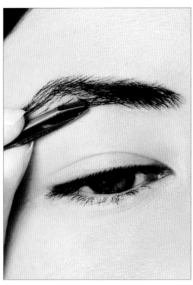

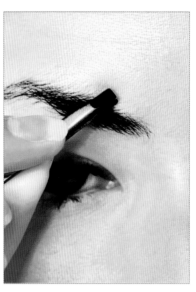

Use flat-head tweezers on very thick brows to get a firm grip. I like to start by tweezing stray hairs on the bridge of the nose.

Next, clean up stray hairs underneath the brow, which can make the lid look too heavy.

A lot of people don't clean up the stray hairs above the brow line, but it's important.

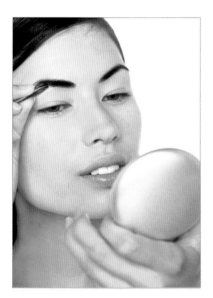

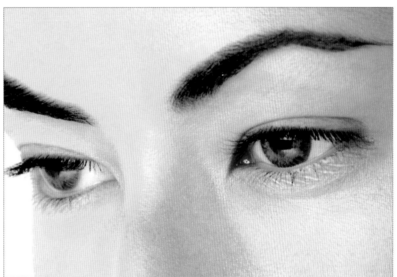

Tweeze your brows in natural light, and use a magnifying mirror if you have one.

The big finish: beautifully shaped and arched brows.

THE BIG TWEEZE

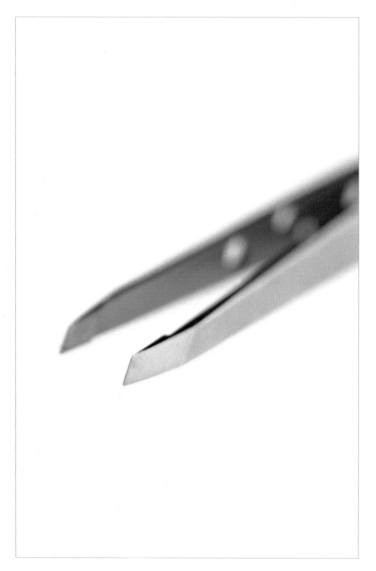

Angle-tipped tweezers like the Rubis Swiss Tweeze are great for grabbing fine hairs.

Follow these instructions for the best results:

✳ Clean your instruments with a little Sea Breeze or alcohol applied to a tissue.

✳ Brush your brows up above the brow line and determine which areas need attention: under the brow line, toward the bridge of the nose, at the end of the eyebrow.

✳ Apply a little moisturizer to soften the brows or tweeze just after getting out of the shower.

✳ Using one swift movement, tweeze hairs in the direction that they grow to avoid breakage.

✳ Pluck only one hair at a time to avoid bare spots in the brow line—this is where a good magnifying mirror comes in handy since it will help you see what you're doing.

✳ Dab a little aloe on the brow area to reduce inflammation and redness.

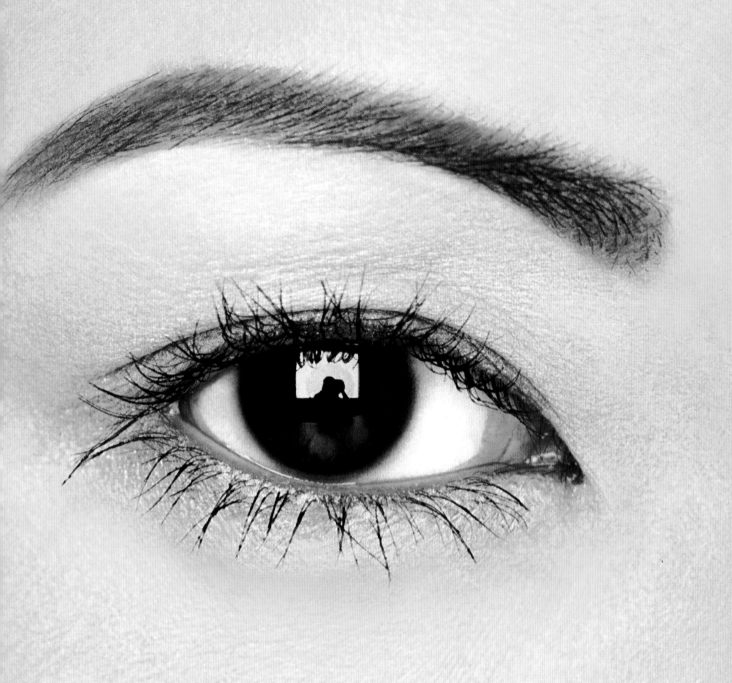

GOOD GROOMING

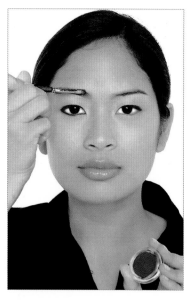

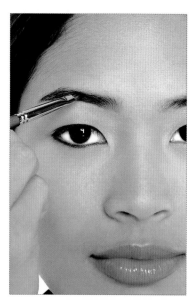

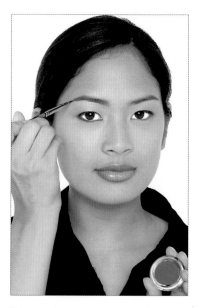

To color your brows and fill in any sparse areas, you'll need a hard angle-tipped brush and a hard dark brown eye shadow.

Starting at the inner corner and working out, apply the powder in short strokes.

If your brows are very short or you've overtweezed in the past, extend the shadow out to create a little more length at the tip.

If your brows are unusually thick or unruly, ask an esthetician to trim them for you. Brushing the brows up above the brow line and trimming the excess can strengthen their shape. This is not something you want to do yourself since removing too much length could just make coarse brows jut out from the face.

If you love the shape of your brows and don't have any gaps to fill in, just brush and go. I'm not a big fan of eyebrow fixatives for Asian women. It's been my experience that they work best on finer brows.

Brows are softer today and have more color. That's why I prefer powders to pencils. The results are just a lot more natural. Besides, pencils are usually limited to a couple of basic shades while powders offer a whole range of colors. Select a shade that's close to your brow's natural color, then add another shade to define or highlight. Choose from fine-spun powder created specifically for eyebrows or hard-pressed eye shadow. You'll also need a good, hard, angle-tipped eyebrow brush that isn't too wide.

I've spent years perfecting my technique for creating beautiful brows, and now I want to share it with you:

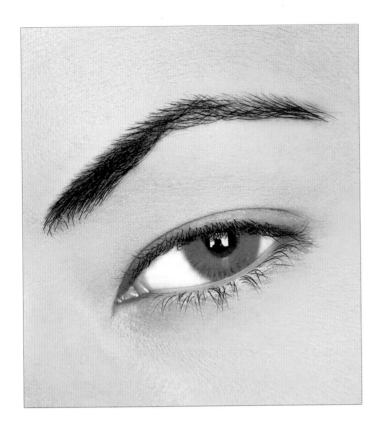

* Prime your canvas by applying foundation to the eyebrow—it helps the powder adhere better.

* If you color your hair, you might want to mix two shades of powder so your brows look more realistic.

* Tweezing gives Asian brows a more precise look.

* Dot the powder onto the brow with the tip of your brush.

* Stroke the powder on in the direction the hair grows.

* Use your eyebrow brush to blend the color.

HOT TIP

If you're having trouble shaping your own brows because you can't see a thing without your glasses, invest in a good magnifying mirror.

HOT TIP

The best place to tweeze your brows is in the car. The rearview mirror lets you get up close and personal, almost like a magnifying mirror would, while daylight puts every stray hair sharply in focus. Please make sure you do this in a car parked in a safe spot.

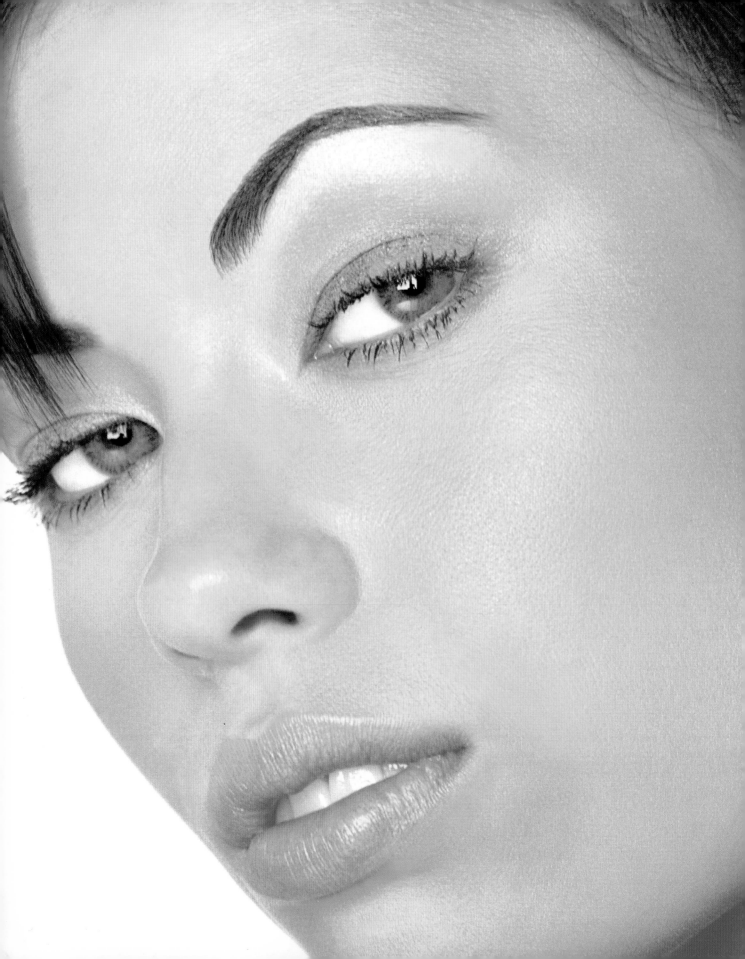

CLASSIC BROW SHAPES

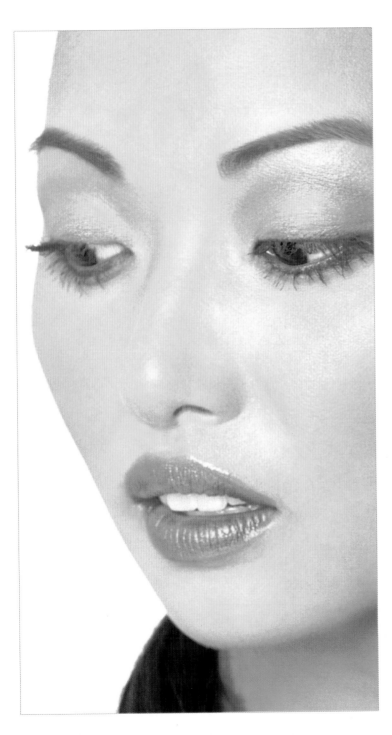

ARCHED: Starts out thick at the inner end, gradually thins to the arch, then tapers off.

ROUNDED: Thickness remains consistent throughout the arch.

THICK AND NATURAL: If you've got it, flaunt it.

THIN AND SHAPELY: Structured like the arched brow but with softer definition, this shape requires a lot of upkeep.

Rounded brows.
FACING PAGE: Classic arched brows.

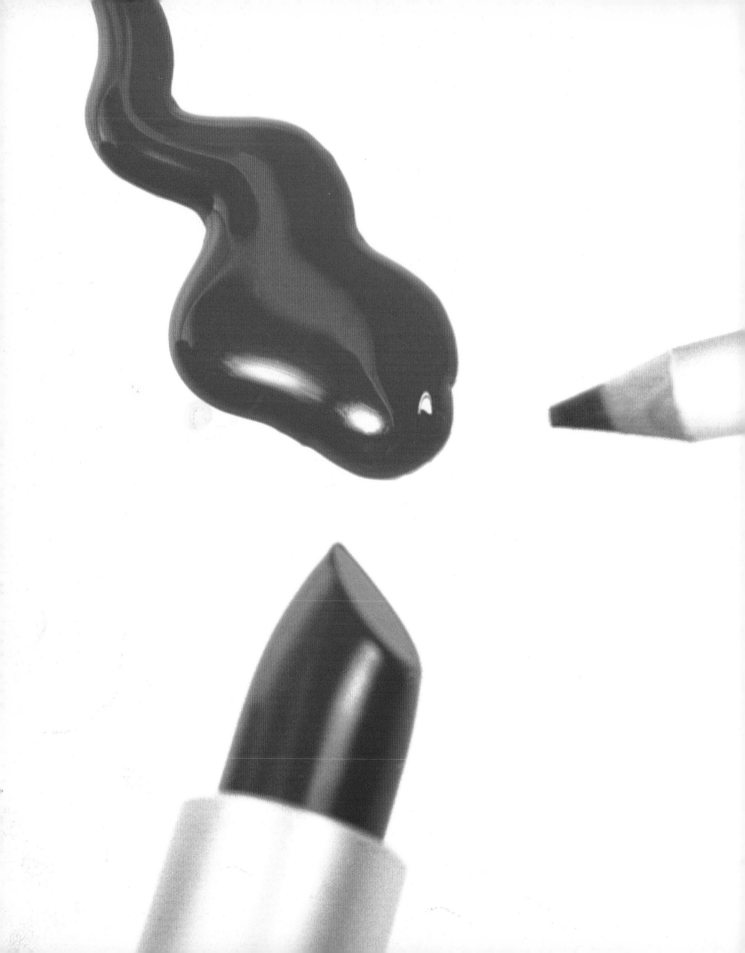

7
LIP SERVICE

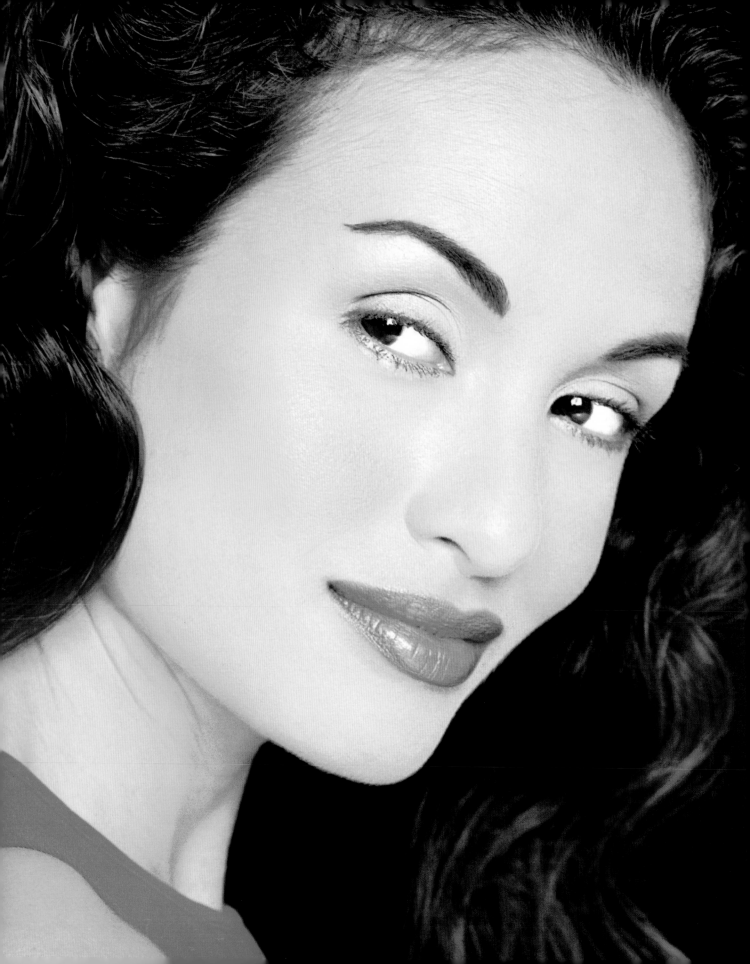

WHETHER YOU PREFER A STRONG RED MOUTH OR JUST A WASH OF COLOR, LIPSTICK IS ONE OF THE EASIEST WAYS TO CREATE A SIGNATURE LOOK. AND SINCE ASIAN WOMEN IN GENERAL TEND TO HAVE GREAT LIPS—BOTH THE UPPER AND LOWER LIP ARE ABOUT THE SAME SIZE—MY ADVICE IS TO MAKE THE MOST OF THEM. THERE ARE SO MANY LOOKS YOU CAN ACHIEVE WITH THE RIGHT SHADE AND THE RIGHT TOOLS. FOR INSTANCE, I THINK RED LIPS ARE GREAT WITH AN ALMOST-NO-MAKEUP LOOK. WANT TO EMPHASIZE A POUT? DAB A LITTLE

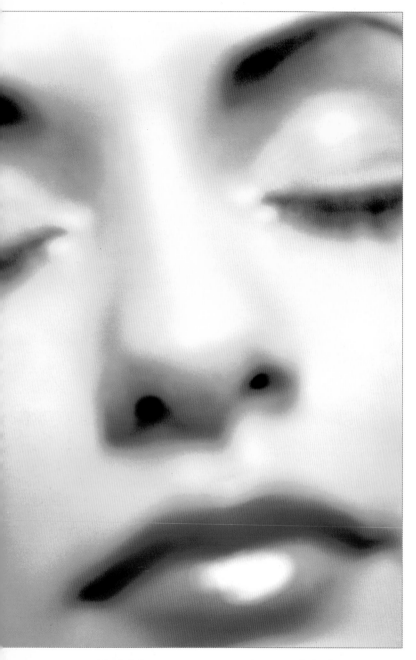

Most Asian women can wear brown-red shades.

frosted lipstick onto the center of the lower lip. Meanwhile, a pale mouth works well with a smoky lid. The idea is to achieve a sense of balance. More important, however, is to blend everything so your lips don't enter the room before you do.

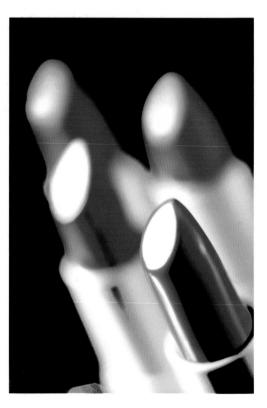

PRIME TIME

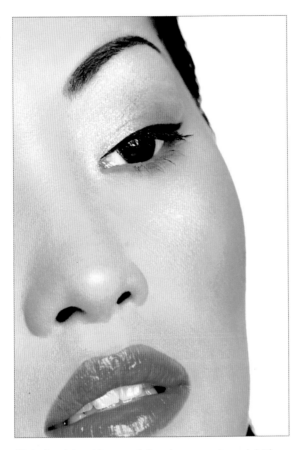

Pink lipstick with a red lip gloss creates nighttime drama.

It's just as important to prime your lips before applying lipstick as it is to prime the skin before applying make-up. Think moist and dewy, not dry and chapped. One of the easiest ways to exfoliate the lips is to rub them vigorously with a bath towel after washing your face or getting out of the shower. When the lips are wet, there's less chance of tearing the skin or causing the lips to bleed. You can also brush your lips with a soft bristle toothbrush to remove dead skin. Some companies have created exfoliating creams specifically for the lips. Lip balms with beeswax or botanical essences will help soothe and protect the lips, but a thin coat of petroleum jelly does the trick as well. At bedtime when you're applying night cream or moisturizer, slather a little on your lips too.

Nutmeg lip gloss adds warmth to this look.

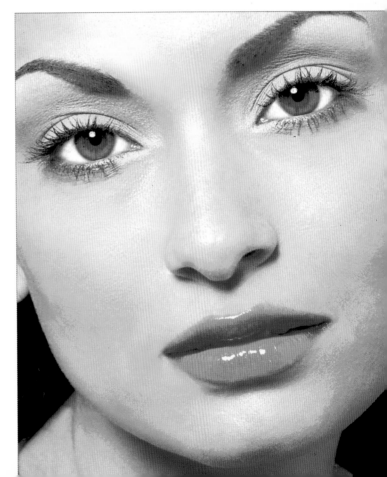

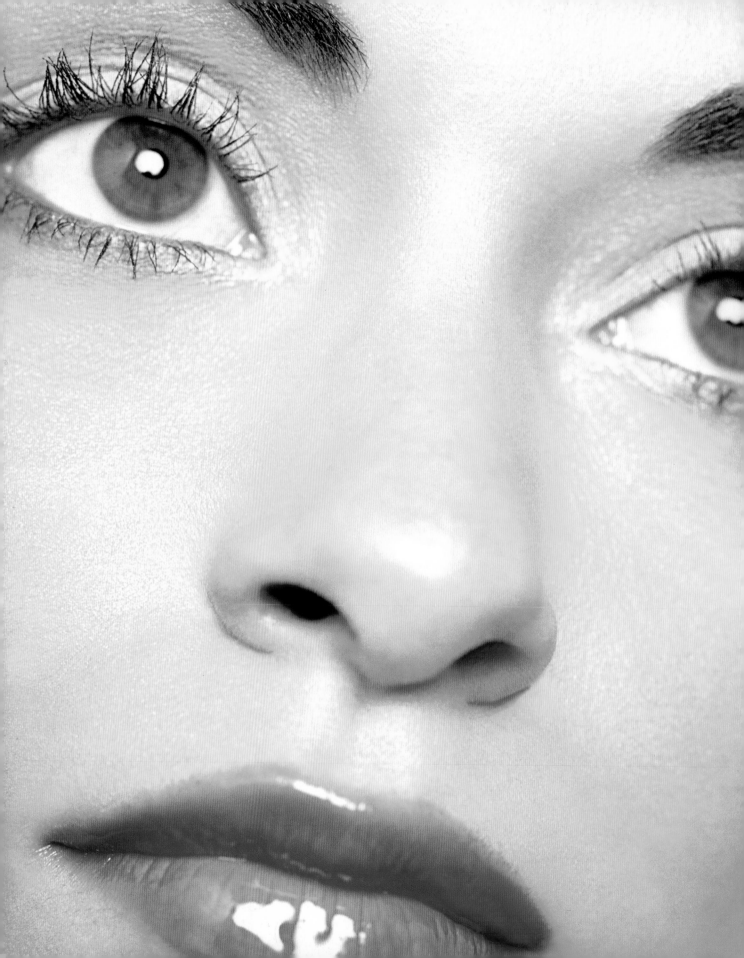

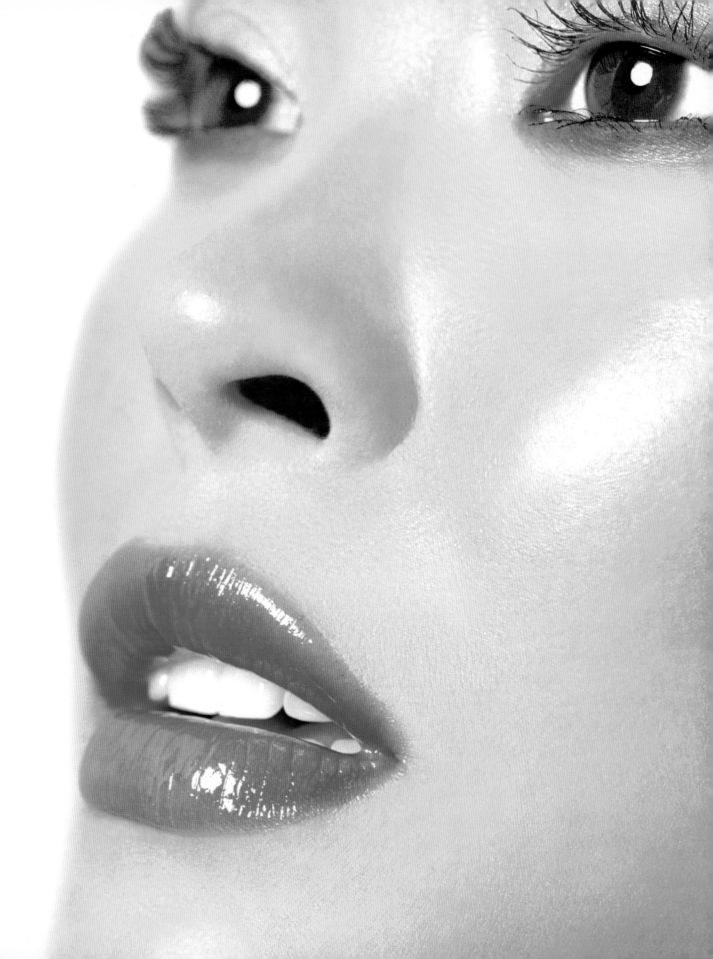

PUCKER UP

There are so many different formulas to choose from that it's important to know which one to use in each situation. These guidelines should help demystify the process:

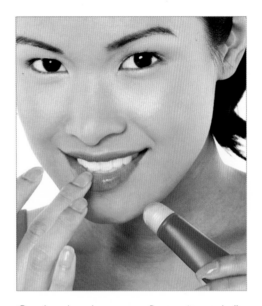

Go ahead and use your fingers to apply lip gloss from a tube.

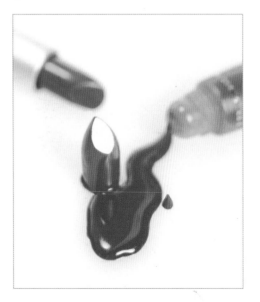

MATTE: Provides a very flat, opaque look. Mixed with a little lip gloss (mattes are the least emollient of all the formulas), they can be ultraglamorous for evening. Still, I don't recommend them for women with very dry or chapped lips.

CREAM: Good coverage but more emollient than mattes, they're great when you want a strong mouth.

SHEER: Translucent coverage with very little pigment. Young women wear them well, but they may make mature women who need a bit more color look washed out. One option: intensify the pigment by blending them with lip pencil.

FROST: Shimmery rather than creamy coverage that reflects the light. Contrary to popular opinion, mature women can wear frosted lipstick. It all depends on the shade and texture. Great for creating the illusion of a fuller lower lip when used with a cream—just dab a little onto the center of the lip. The nighttime is always the right time for frosted shades.

STAINS: Literally soaks into the lips, leaving just a hint of color. Since stains tend to be drying, moisturize your lips well before using them.

LIP GLOSS: Comes in pots—for sanitary reasons use a lip brush to apply it—or tubes. Can be worn alone or mixed with mattes, stains, and pencils for a creamier look.

PENCIL IT IN

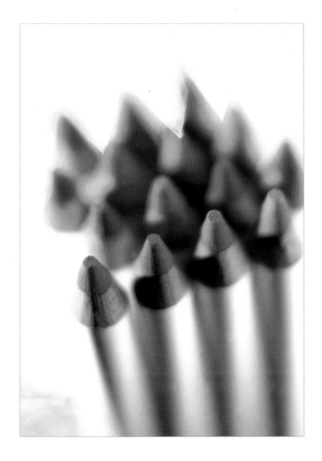

Generally I don't recommend using lip pencils. What I've discovered is that most people tend to choose the wrong shade (too light or too dark for the lipstick they're wearing) or they go overboard, creating a shape that's unnatural. The biggest faux pas: using a dark pencil with a lighter shade of lipstick. Still, there are a few exceptions to this rule:

✳ Lip pencils can provide a base to intensify the pigment in sheer or translucent shades. The trick is to use a firm-tipped lip brush to "smudge the line" and work the color into the lips.

✳ Create the illusion of a fuller upper or lower lip by coloring just slightly outside the lip line. Again, remember to blend.

✳ Lining the lips keeps red lipstick from creeping into tiny lines around the mouth.

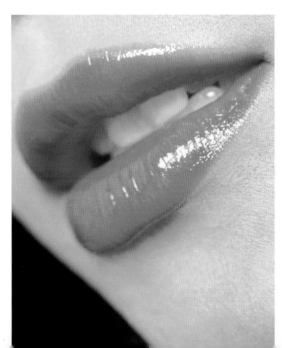

1

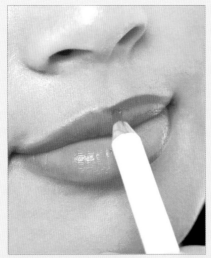

Lip liner helps to keep lipstick from bleeding.

2

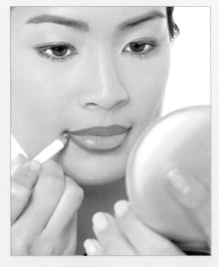

Choose a lip liner shade that closely matches your lipstick.

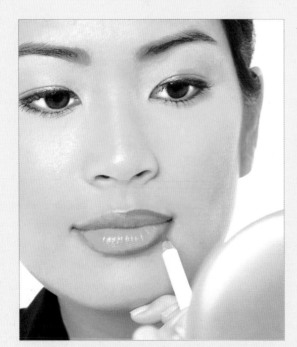

It's best to follow your natural lip line.

3

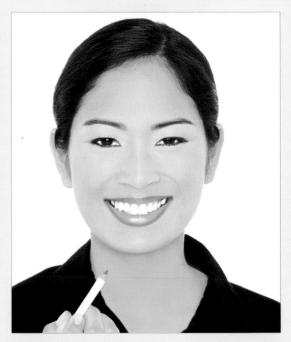

Lips that are lined and defined.

4

RED ALERT

Red lips are the hardest to do well. The contrast against lighter skin magnifies every mistake. If you don't have a steady hand, use a lip pencil to outline your lips first, then fill them in with lipstick and blend everything together with a latex sponge. It's also important to choose the right shade of red for your skin tone and hair color.

BLUE-REDS: The majority of Asian women with dark hair and olive to fair skin can wear these shades.

ORANGE-REDS: Most Asian women can wear them, but they can make pale olive skin look sallow.

BROWN-REDS: Again, most Asian women can wear them.

PINK-REDS: Not recommended for most Asian women, but Eurasian or Amerasian women with very pale skin can carry them off.

RED LIPSTICK
SAYS GLAMOUR TO ME.
IT'S ALWAYS A SAFE
BET FOR EVENING.

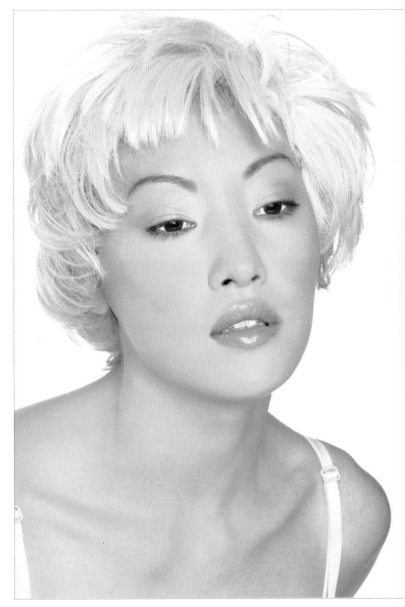

Bleached blonde hair and iridescent pink gloss are pure sex kitten.

THE RULES

✳ Don't use a dark lip pencil with a lighter shade of lipstick.

✳ Blend everything. You don't want your lips to enter the room before you do.

✳ A stronger lip balances a nearly nude eye.

✳ Smoky eyes require a paler mouth.

✳ Use a lip brush to apply color. It helps you create a more precise shape and distributes the pigment evenly.

✳ A latex sponge is an important tool. Use it to blend your lipstick—it picks up the excess—so your lips don't look heavy or gooey.

✳ Avoid dark colors if you have thin lips. Instead, highlight the top lip and stick with sheer colors.

✳ Lighter shades create the illusion that small, round lips are larger.

✳ Your makeup isn't finished until your lips are done.

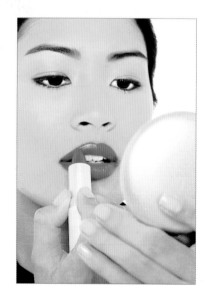

Apply lipstick directly from the tube.

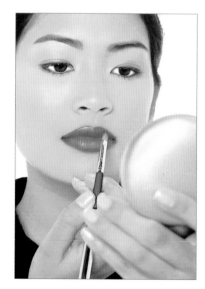

Then go over your lips with a lip brush to create a more precise line.

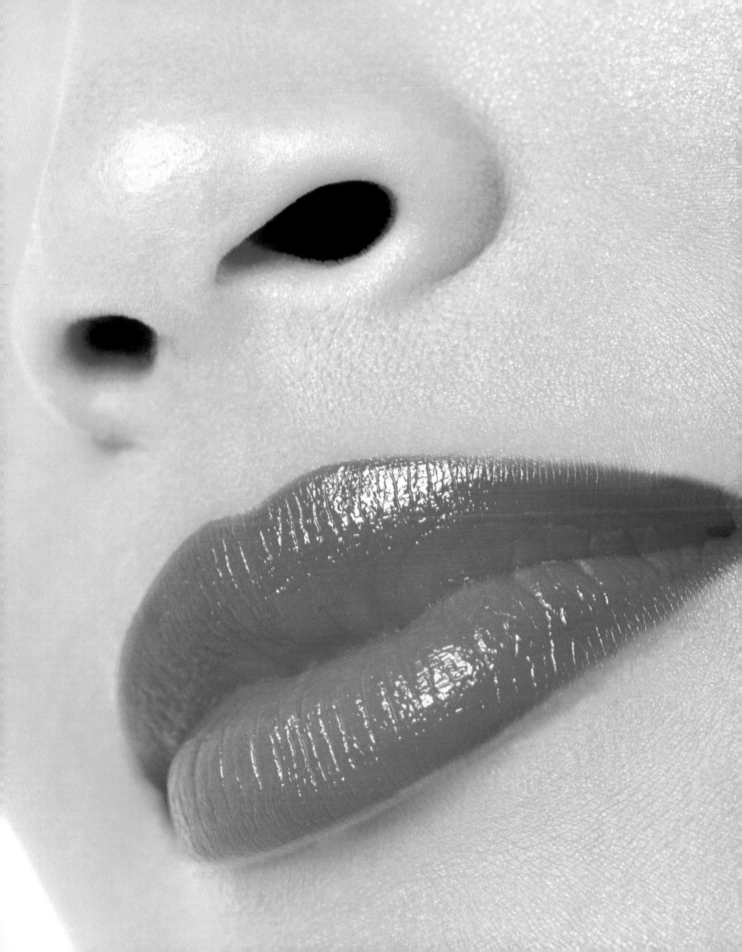

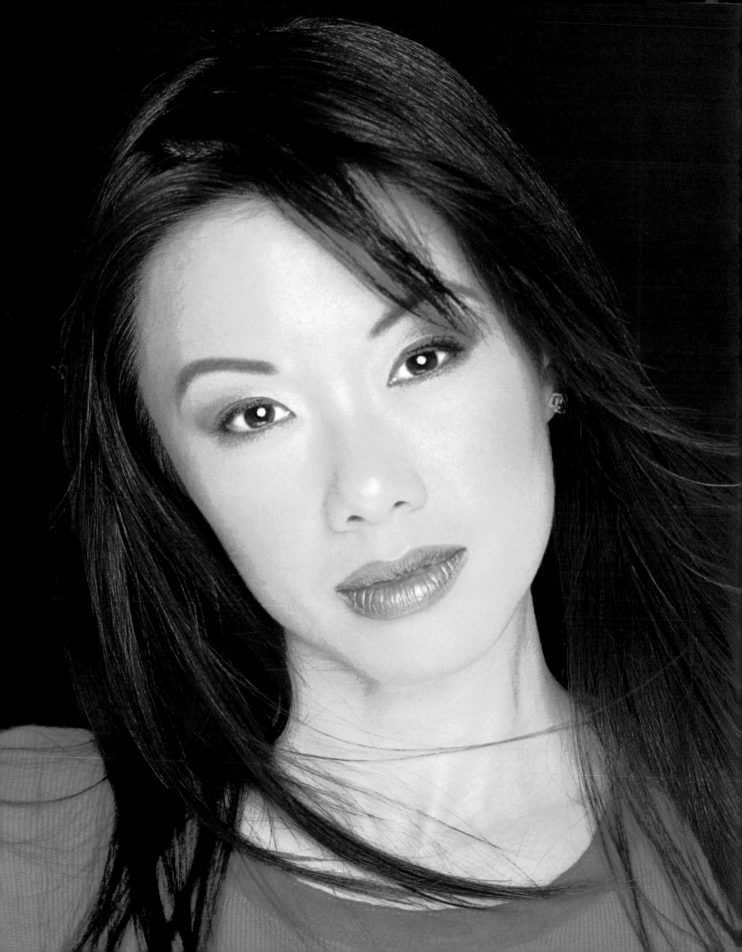

8

ROLE MODELS

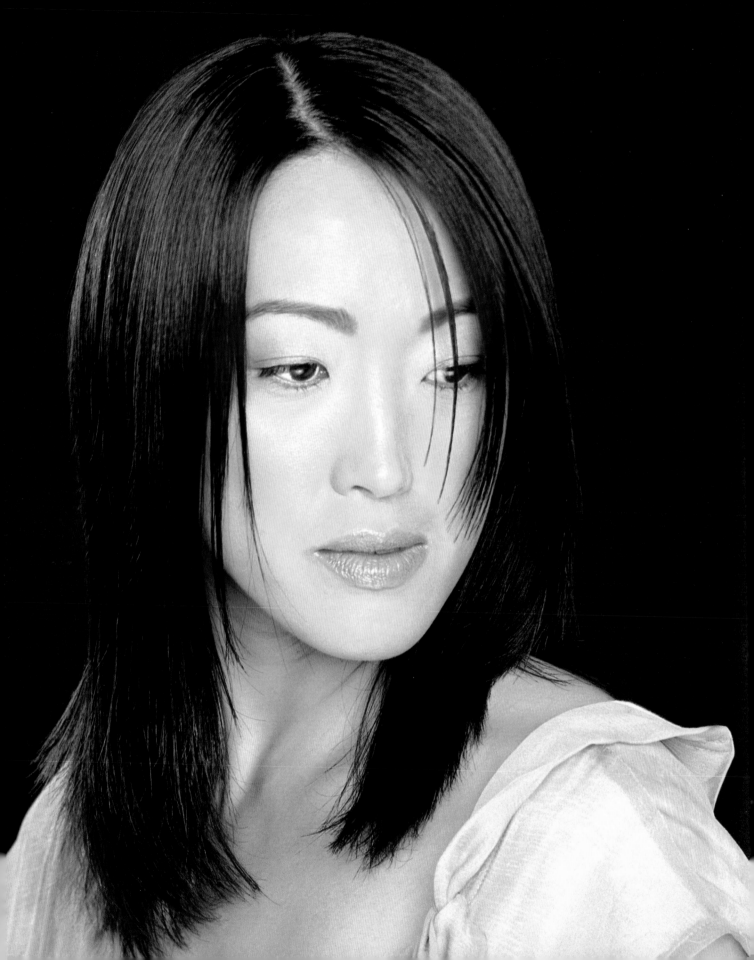

EVERY WOMAN IN THIS CHAPTER IS A ROLE MODEL FOR ME, FROM LISA LING, THE BEAUTIFUL COHOST OF ABC'S *THE VIEW*, TO SHIRLEY TOMIOKA, WHO, AT FORTY, IS ONE OF JAPAN'S TOP DISC JOCKEYS. EACH OF THEM IS REMARKABLY SELF-ASSURED AND POSITIVELY FEARLESS IN THE FACE OF ADVERSITY. THEY ALSO SHARE A STRONG SENSE OF PERSONAL STYLE. MY FRIEND ANN LEWIS, FOR EXAMPLE, IS ABSOLUTELY CRAZY ABOUT LEOPARD PRINTS, SO MUCH SO THAT THEY'VE BECOME HER TRADEMARK. THE FACT THAT THESE WOMEN ALL SEEM TO GET BETTER WITH AGE MAY HAVE MORE TO DO WITH ATTITUDE THAN WITH GENETICS. I'VE NEVER KNOWN ONE OF THEM TO SET LIMITS ON HERSELF. I KNOW HOW IMPORTANT IT IS TO HAVE ROLE MODELS YOU CAN IDENTIFY WITH. I ALSO KNOW HOW FEW THERE HAVE BEEN FOR ASIAN WOMEN UNTIL RECENTLY. IT'S MY HOPE THAT AS YOU TURN THE PAGES YOU'LL SEE YOURSELF IN WOMEN LIKE SHARON TAY OR YU HAYAMI. WHO KNOWS — MAYBE THEIR SUCCESS WILL INSPIRE YOURS.

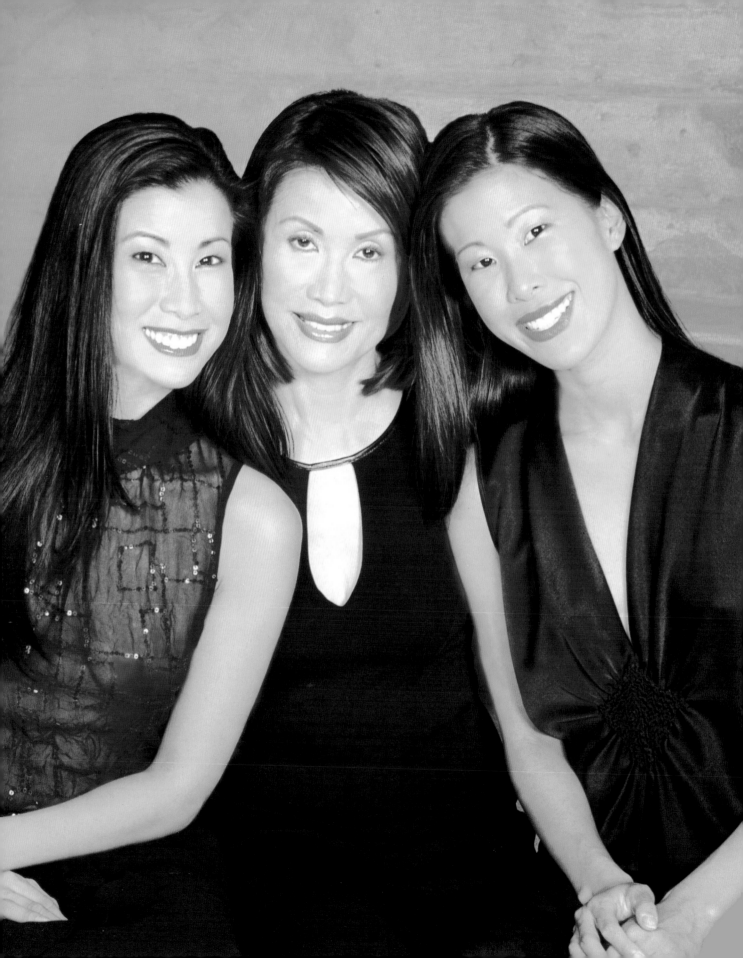

LISA, MARY, AND LAURA LING

Lisa is one of the talented cohosts of ABC's popular daytime talk show *The View*. She was really happy to be part of this book and wanted to be photographed with her mother, Mary, and her sister, Laura. What I love about these women is that they're totally comfortable in their own skins. They are willing to experiment, but they also know that their real power has nothing to do with how much makeup they wear.

Lisa is a contemporary young woman who exudes a lot of inner strength. That's why I chose a strong shade of red lipstick for her. I also wanted to make the most of her beautiful almond-shaped eyes. I started by lining them with a dark powder shadow, then adding some shimmery taupe powder on the outer corner of her eyelid. She really doesn't need much foundation, just a light base I set with dual-finish powder.

Laura is very understated, but she was game for anything. I wanted her to see herself in a new light so I used shades of pink and blue on her eyes and bright fuchsia lip color.

Mary was a whole other story. She's a beautiful woman in her own right, but she's just Mom to Laura and Lisa so I was really grateful when she gave me carte blanche. I felt it was important to do something dramatic so I blended shades of peacock green, khaki, and taupe eye shadow on her eyelids, then used a little gold on the brow bone to open up her eyes. A bronze powder blush shot with gold gave her a radiant glow. A deep shade of bronze lipstick pulled the whole look together. She beamed when she saw herself in the mirror. "I never knew I could wear colors like these," she said.

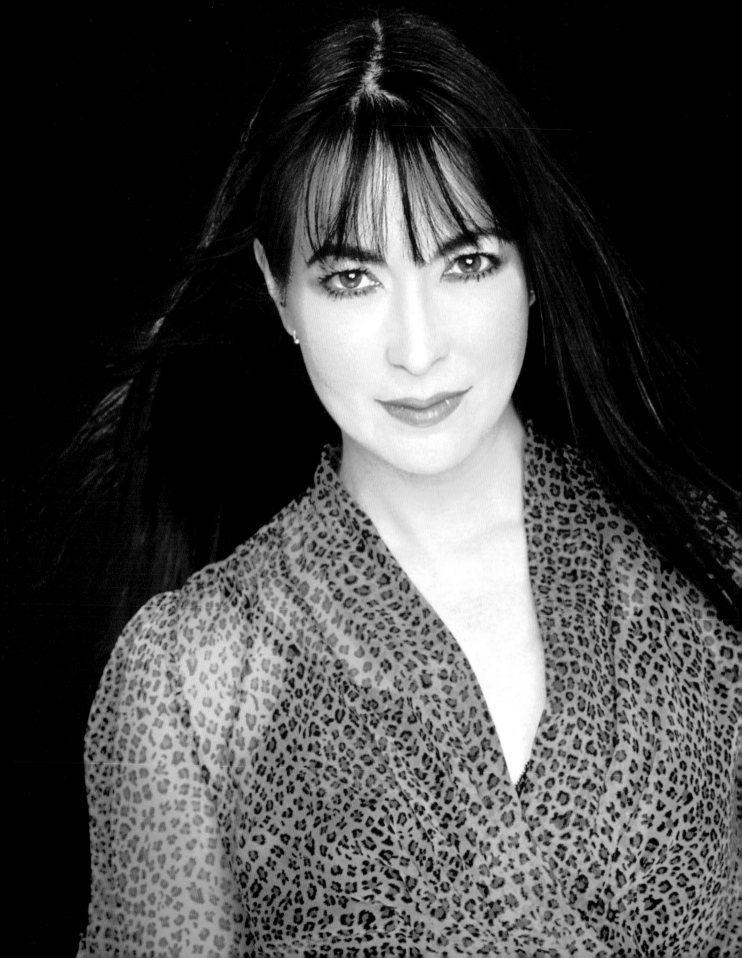

ANN LEWIS

Ann is a musical phenomenon in Japan, a real creative genius. She's recorded forty-three albums during her career, and even after twenty-five years in the limelight she's still considered a style icon. We've been friends for years, and I've gotten to know her tastes very well. Ann loves leopard prints. They're her trademark. She's also happiest when I give her smoky eyes. It's part of her personality, so why fight it? Ann is pretty enough to carry off the pink and blue eye shadow I used on Lisa Ling, but she wouldn't feel comfortable in it. She's not a big fan of blush either so I just used a little, kind of a soft, buttery-pink shade. To further soften the effect, I dipped my blusher brush into some loose powder first, then into the blush. A little lipstick in a soft shade of rose completed her look.

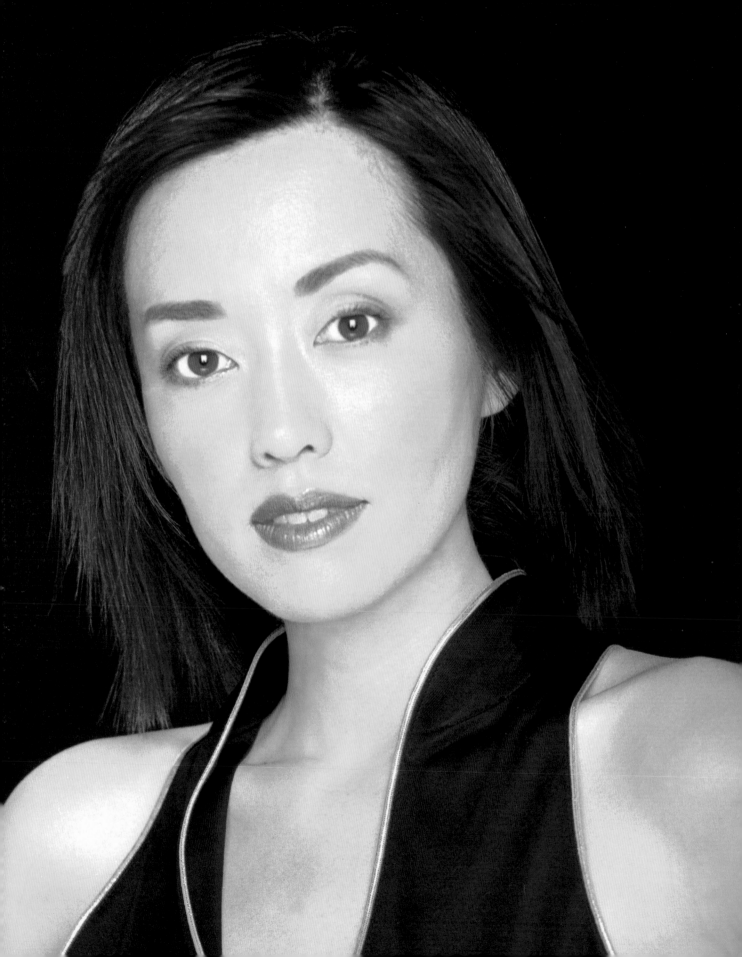

YU HAYAMI

Yu is another close friend of mine, someone I've always thought of as a little sister even though she's only a year younger than me. She's a talented actress and singer who has starred in numerous plays, films, and TV shows in Japan. I hadn't seen her for a while, but when she came to sit for this photo I noticed right away that there was something different about her. It was as if she had crossed some threshold and had come into her own as a woman. And that's precisely what I wanted to capture on film.

Yu's eyes are deep-set, so the Shadows and Light technique really worked on her. To give her a very wide-eyed look, I used highlighter powder on the inner part of her eyelids and a darker, shimmery shade of bronze on the outer part of her eyelids. She has great cheekbones, which I enhanced with a dusting of powder blush mixed with a little loose powder. I applied a shade of deep topaz lipstick, then added a little gold gloss on top to create a little extra shimmer. The result: a look that's refined and elegant, glamorous yet simple.

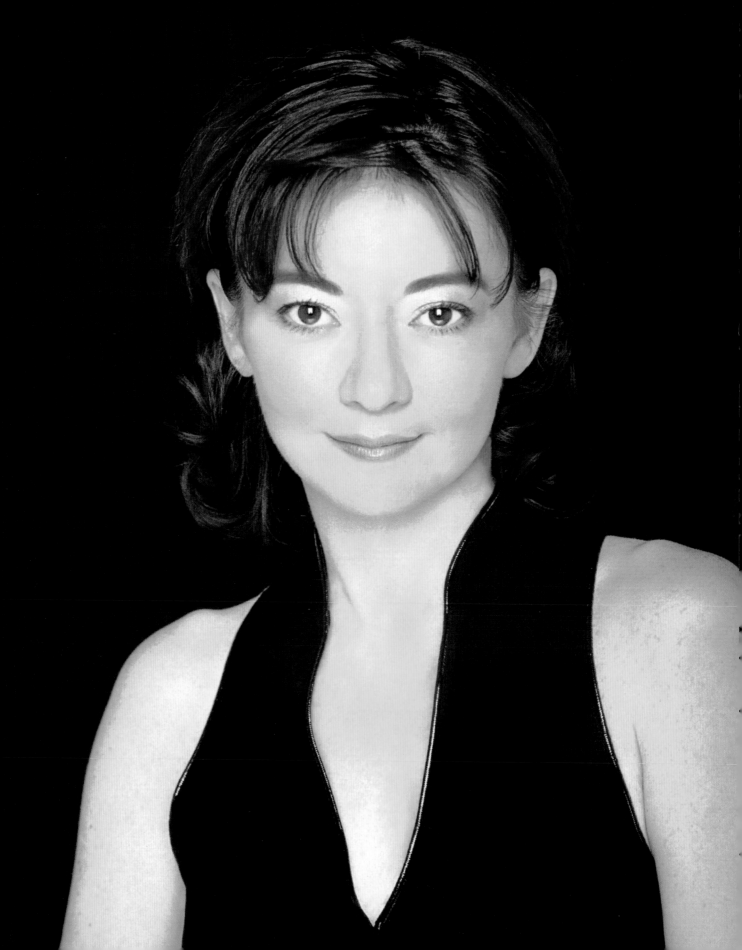

SHIRLEY TOMIOKA

At forty, Shirley is one of Japan's top deejays. Since she's normally just a disembodied voice, I wanted to create a personality for her. Shirley is definitely young at heart and she keeps up with trends, but she was in a rut when it came to makeup. In fact, she wears very little. I deliberately chose colors she would never think of wearing, like teal blue and pink eye shadow. Again, I used the Shadows and Light technique to bring out her eyes. I felt that heavy eyeliner would have been overkill so I just used a little teal shadow around her eyes instead. I also went with a vibrant shade of coral lipstick. When she looked in the mirror, she was pleasantly surprised at the result. I think it boosted her confidence. She looked really modern, but I was able to bring out another side of her—a young, sophisticated side that she tends to hide.

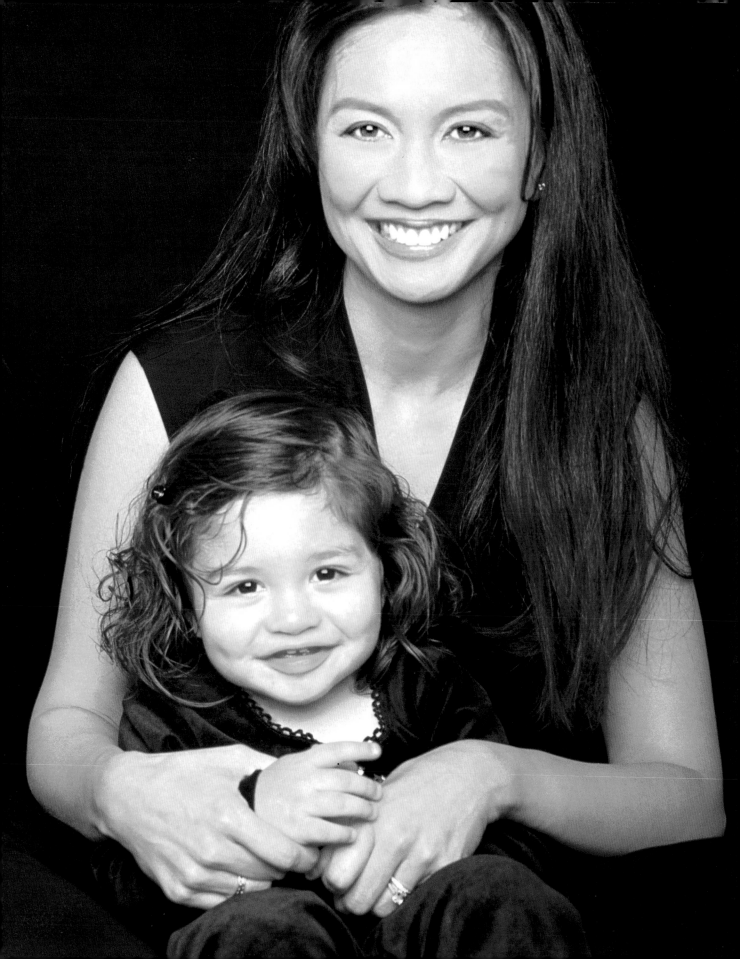

EMILY AND JORDAN GOLDSTEIN

Emily and her husband, Mark, own several Madison & EmmaGold Boutiques in Los Angeles, where they sell hip, high-end designer clothing. Emily is one of those amazing women who seem to have it all. She's a wife, a mother, and a successful businesswoman. Because Emily is a natural beauty and has such a playful spirit, I wanted to photograph her with her daughter Jordan, who's two and already has her mother's spectacular cheekbones. With a face like Emily's, less is definitely more when it comes to makeup so I took a minimalist approach—neutral eye shadow, soft mocha/pink lipstick—but I played up her biggest assets. I used a really dark shade of mascara to bring out her lashes, which are naturally long and lush. Then I applied a little nutmeg powder blush to the apples of her cheeks since they're so prominent.

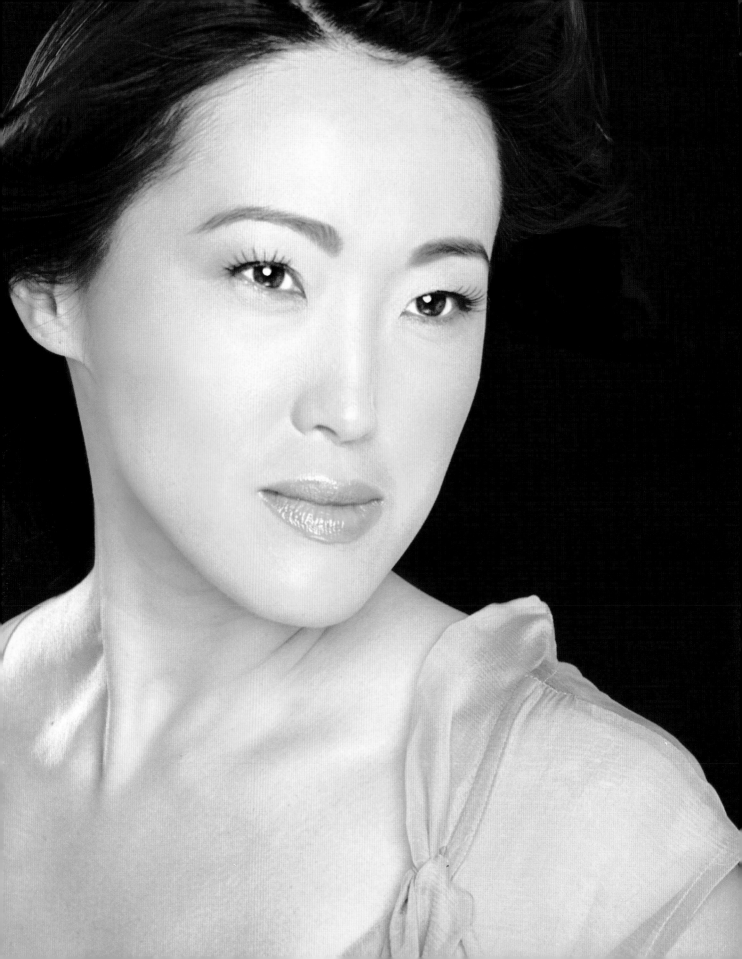

JOOMI HA

Joomi is a retired high-fashion model with two teenage sons. She's one of those ageless beauties who really make me look forward to my forties. Joomi has an absolutely flawless complexion, and I wanted to make the most of it. I used a very luminous foundation to create a lot of reflection. She wore a beautiful dress, very soft and feminine in shades of coral and lime green. It inspired me to use similar colors on her eyes. I used a soft gold shade of eye shadow on the inner part of her eyelid to bring out her eyes, then used a coral shade on the outer part of her eyelid. I also added a few individual lashes to play up her mysterious eyes. Finally, I mixed a little nude lip gloss with some opalescent pure pigment. Joomi seems very vulnerable to me, almost shy being in front of the camera again, and I think you get a sense of that here.

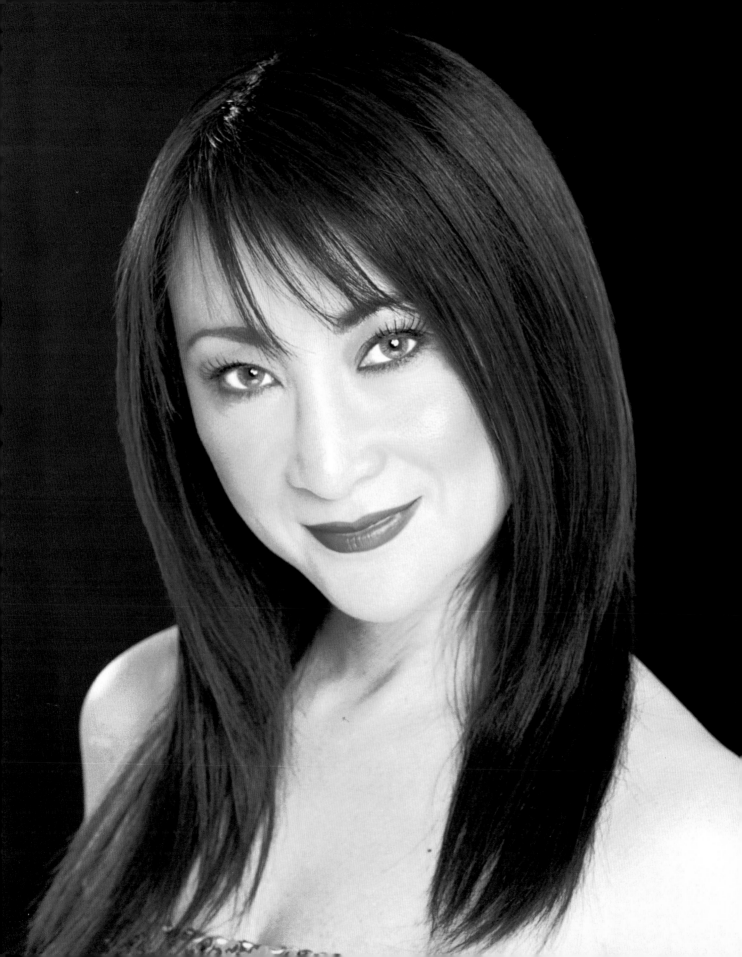

JEANNIE HARTH

Jeannie is another one of those forty-something women who seem to get better with age. I think it has a lot to do with her willingness to take chances. She's also smart, and it shows. Jeannie is a fashion designer/stylist, and she set the tone for the whole session when she breezed into the studio, picked out a skirt she loved, and proceeded to wear it as a dress. That's when I knew that I could get as flamboyant as I wanted. A woman this self-confident could pull anything off. I gave her a strong mouth—cranberry lip gloss over cranberry lipstick. I worked with several shades of eye shadow, blending soft lavender and dark pink on her top lid, then working a little pearl highlighter up onto her brow bone. Finally, I lined her eyes with a dark charcoal powder shadow and added a few individual lashes.

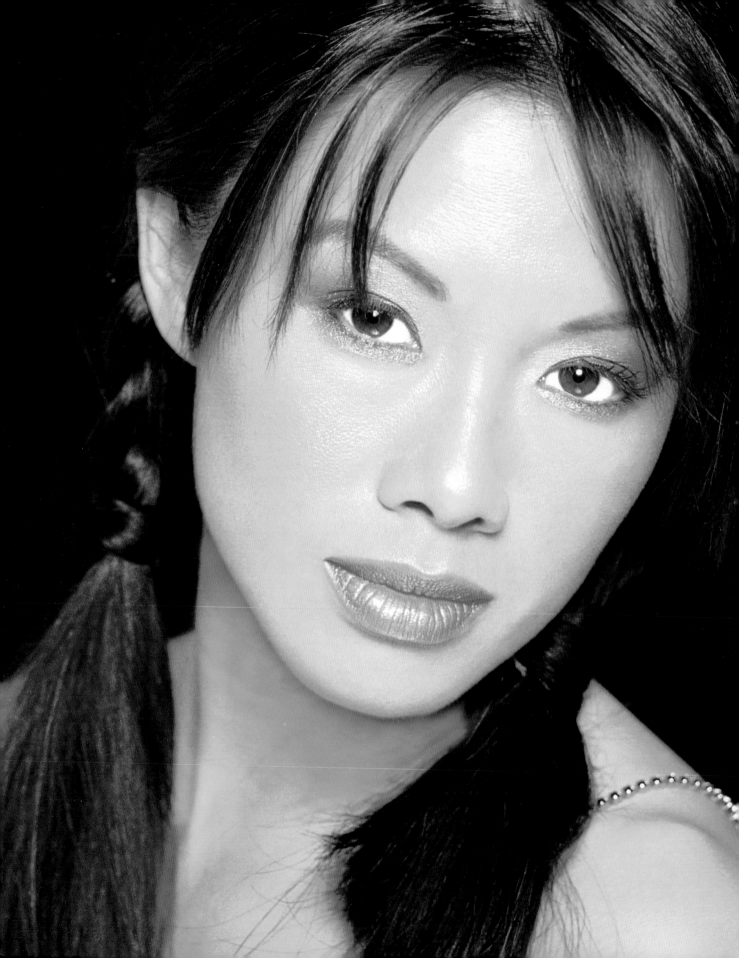

SHARON TAY

Sharon is an anchorwoman on KTLA-TV in Los Angeles, which means she has to maintain a pretty conservative look. But she's also very sensual, and that's what I wanted to bring out. It's a side of her the public never sees. For me, lip gloss with a touch of gold literally oozes sensuality. I also liked the idea of sticking to neutral shades of brown and pearl eye shadow, then lining her eyes with a soft brown powder shadow. Even though she was born in Singapore, Sharon is a real California girl who sports a year-round tan. Fortunately she has great skin so I was able to use a sheer foundation in a warm shade that matched her skin tone. To set her foundation, I chose a bronzing powder instead of a translucent powder to enhance her healthy glow. Finally, I used a few individual lashes to open up her eyes. She loved them. In fact, when she looked in the mirror, she said, "Wow! I really look Asian." Mission accomplished.

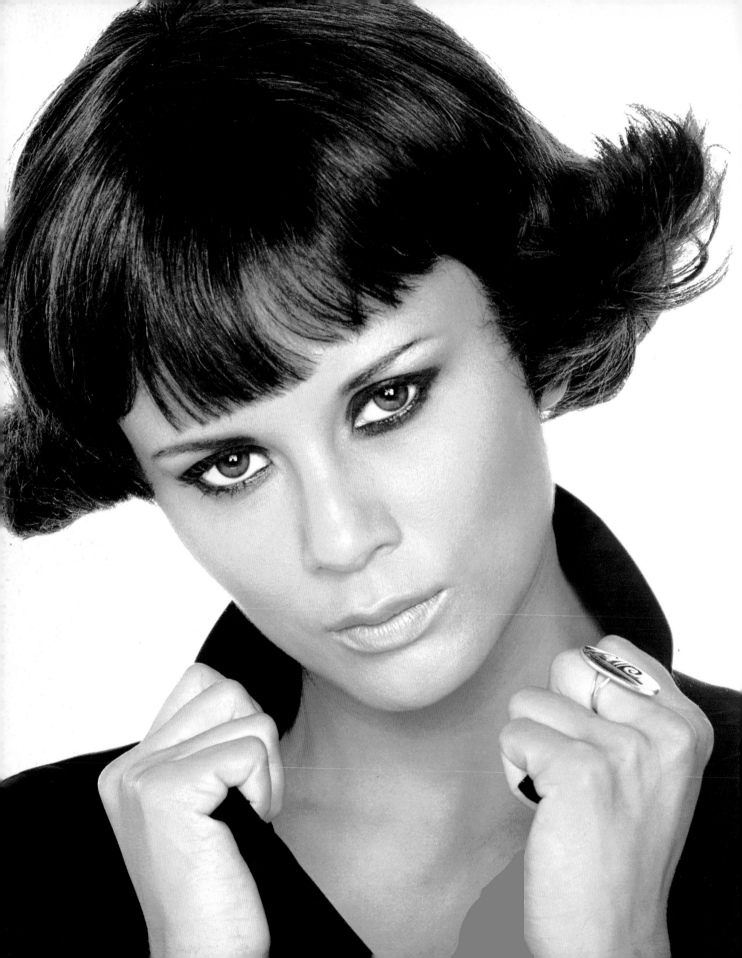

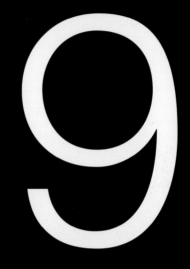

MAKEOVERS

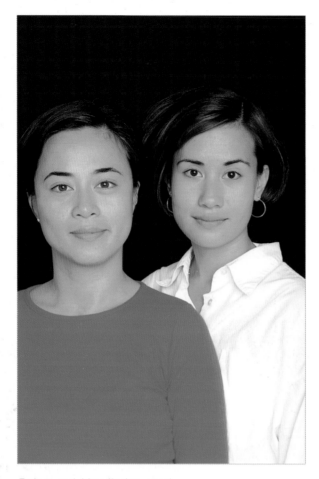

Before and After (facing page)

RIA & THERESE

Ria and Therese are sisters, and while they look very much alike, their personalities are quite different. Ria, who's almost eight years older than Therese, is a very nurturing person and very wise. I decided right away that I wanted to play up those qualities. I started by applying a creamy foundation that provided slightly heavier coverage, for a truly flawless complexion. I went with shimmery earth tones on her eyes and a strong metallic shade of red lipstick that makes her look sophisticated and underlines her maturity. Therese, on the other hand, is a very independent young woman, very smart, but she's still got a youthful innocence, almost a naiveté. Consequently, everything about her makeup is light and airy. Her foundation is very luminous, almost transparent. I used cheek gel instead of powder blush and a sheer cranberry shade of lip gloss instead of lipstick. It's really just a wash of color, but it's perfect for someone her age. To me, both sisters look absolutely beautiful, yet there's never any doubt that each is her own person.

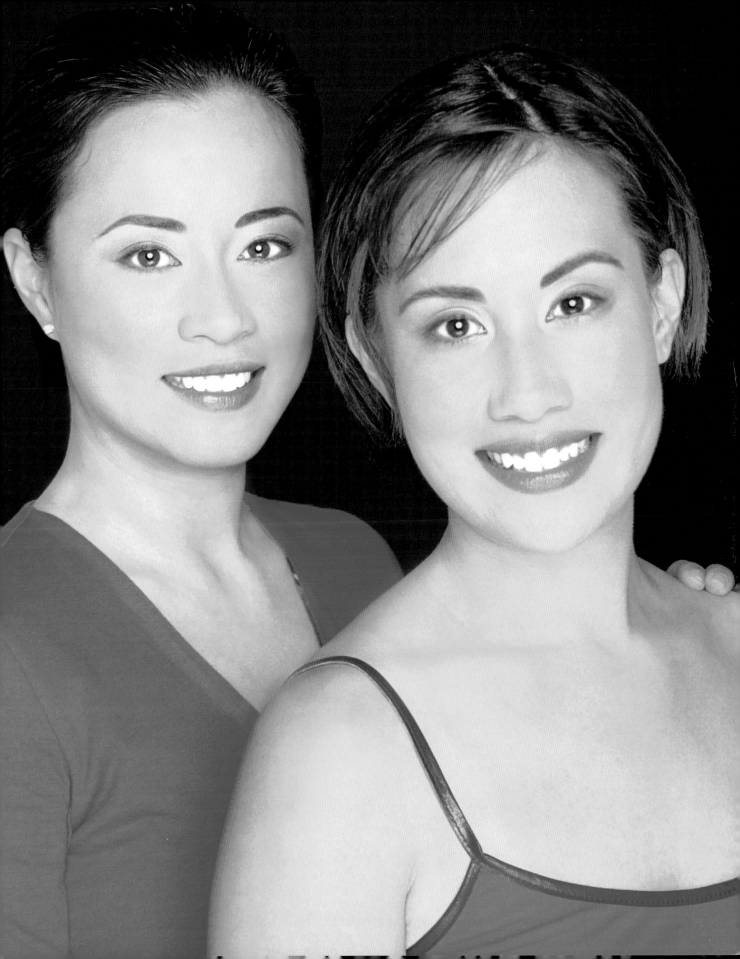

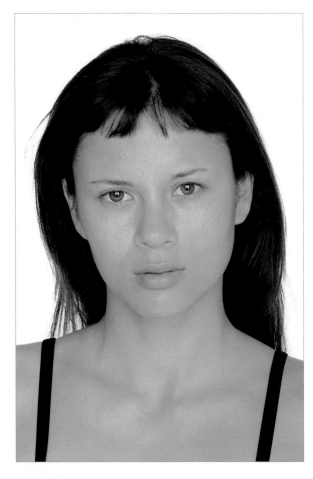

Before and After (facing page)

MIRJAM

Mirjam (pronounced Miriam) is Swiss, Dutch, and Indonesian, with a gorgeous peaches-and-cream complexion with yellow undertones. To balance out her skin tone, I chose a foundation with a yellow base—remember my rule about how you can never have too much yellow in your foundation. Then to counterbalance the warm tones in the foundation, I used cool, pastel shades of pink and lavender eye shadow and a deep cranberry shade of lipstick. One of Mirjam's best features in her beautiful oval-shaped face, which I played up with a shimmery highlight powder. To even out her brows, which she had over-tweezed, I used a stiff, angle-tipped brush to fill them in with a little dark brown powder shadow.

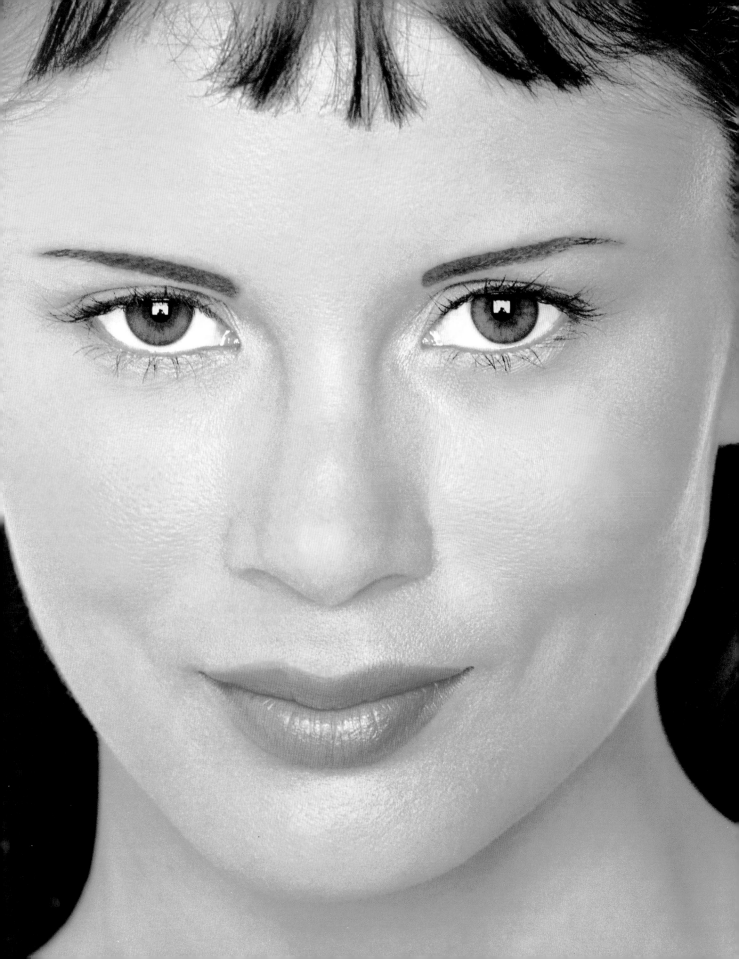

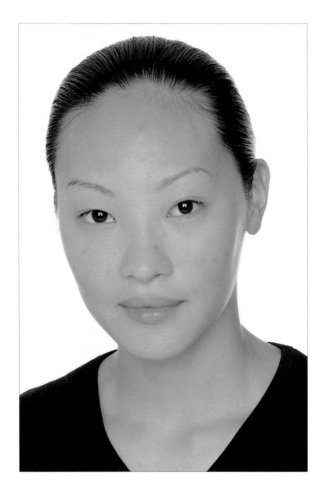

Before and After (facing page)

ELLIE

Ellie, who is in her early twenties, is Korean. She's got really beautiful Asian features and killer brows. Her skin has a tendency to break out, so the first thing I did was concentrate on evening out her skin tone and creating a flawless finish. First I spot-treated any blemishes with concealer. Then I applied a good strong base of cake foundation. Finally, I went over her entire face with a latex sponge and my dual-finish powder. After that, all I had to do was play up her eyes and lips. Since her eyes are small and close-set, I wanted to create the illusion that they were bigger and farther apart than they are so I smudged the outer edges only with a dark coffee-brown powder liner. Warm shades of coral on her eyes and lips make her look as natural as possible.

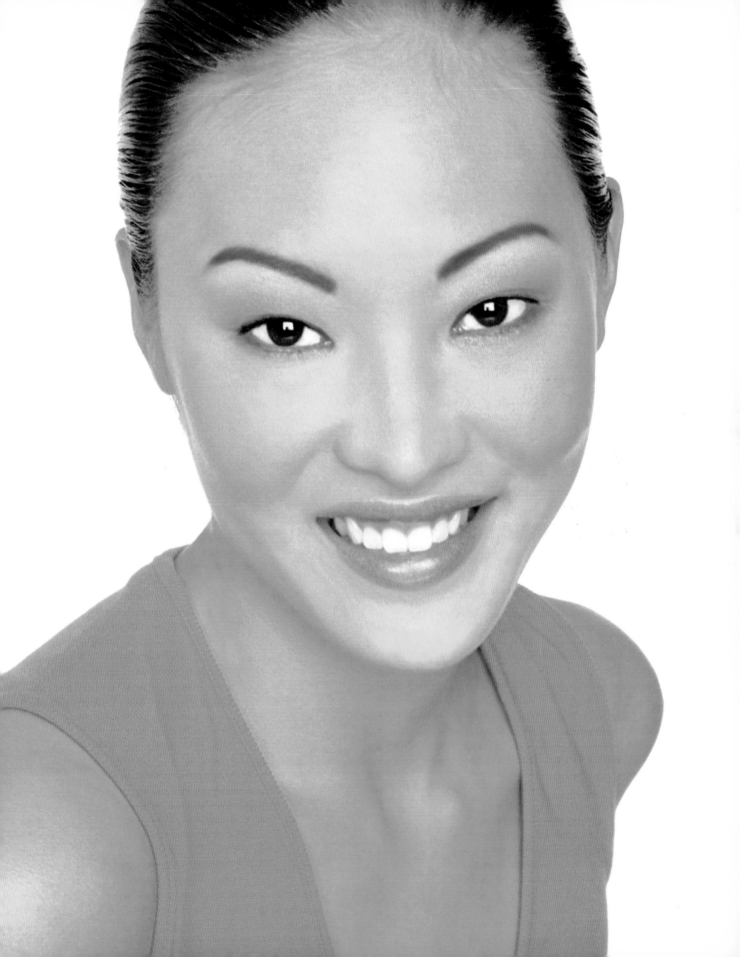

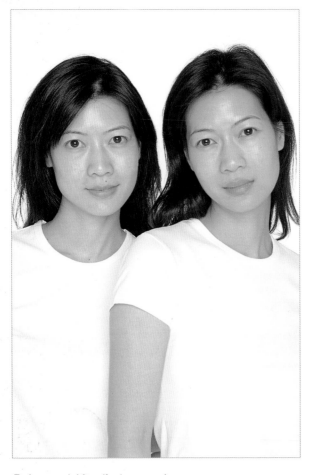

Before and After (facing page)

ARLENE & ADA

Arlene and Ada are identical twins, but that's where the similarity ends. Arlene is really outgoing, while Ada is shy. But instead of playing up their differences, I decided it would be fun to use cosmetics to call attention to the fact that they look so much alike. It's the cosmetic equivalent of dressing them in matching outfits. Since they were both wearing such dark dresses, I didn't want their makeup to look too harsh. Ultimately I settled on a very natural, almost neutral look—soft earth tones on the eyes, a bit stronger mouth.

One thing I was sure about was that I wanted to draw attention to their beautiful milky-white skin. One of my favorite ways to cause light to refract off a surface is to add a little luminescent base to my regular foundation, which is what I did here. Then I set everything with a light dusting of translucent dual-finish powder.

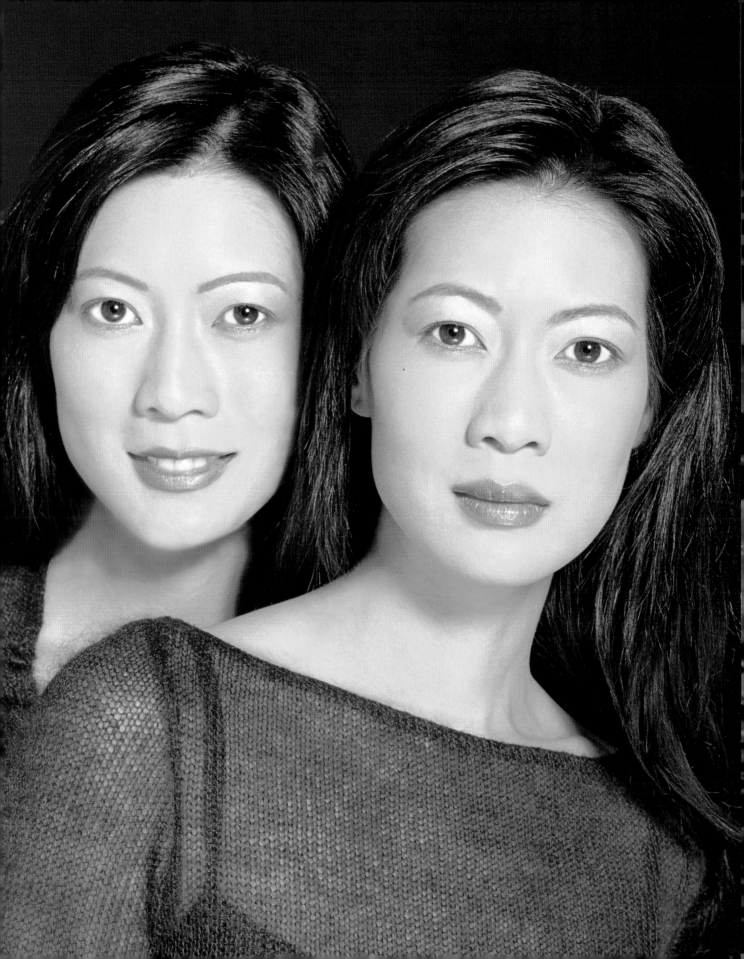

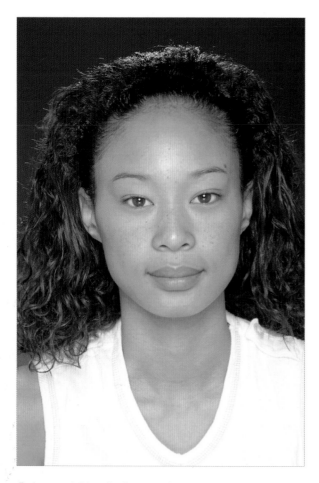

Before and After (facing page)

YOUNG

Young is part Korean, part African-American, which in her case has created an interesting blend of features. Her almond-shaped eyes are definitely Asian, but she also has sensual full lips that are proof of her African-American ancestry. Her biggest beauty challenge, as with many women of mixed race, is finding the right foundation. She actually has a lot of red undertones in her skin, which I tried to counterbalance by using warm tones. Since her features are so distinctive, I didn't want to disguise or overpower them. With women like Young, too much makeup just detracts from their exotic beauty, which is why I decided to take a minimalist approach. First, I cleaned up her brows a bit, then used a soft powder to define their shape. I used a little nutmeg eye shadow on her lid and warm yellow highlighter on her brow bone, then lined her eyes with a soft powder. Since her lips already have a lot of pigment in them, I merely used a little nude lip gloss to add a bit of shimmer and shine.

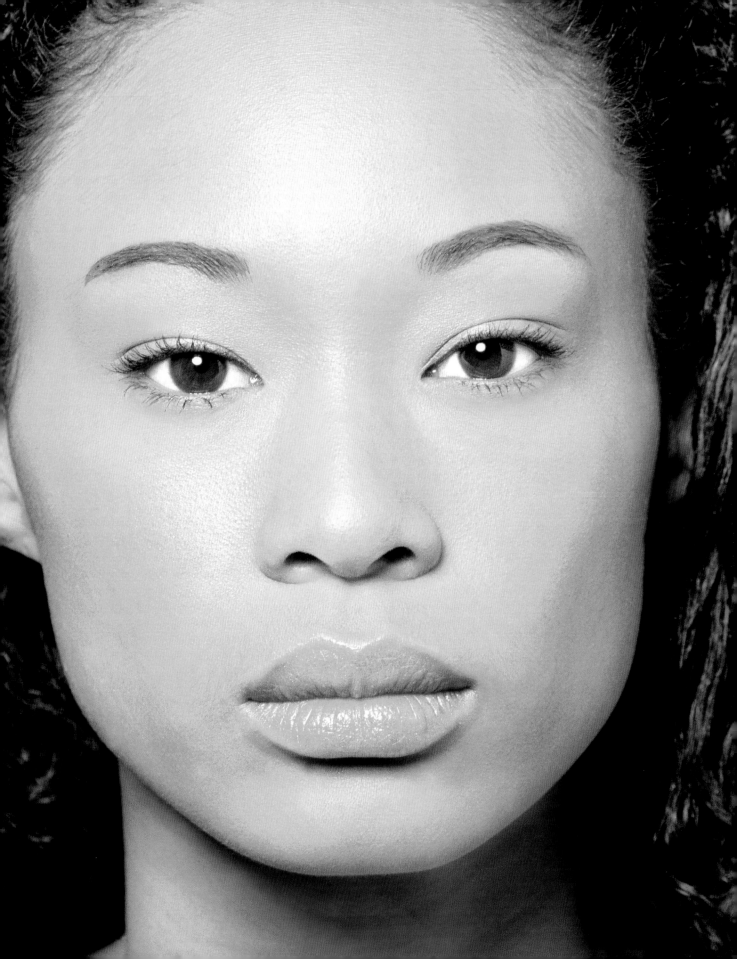

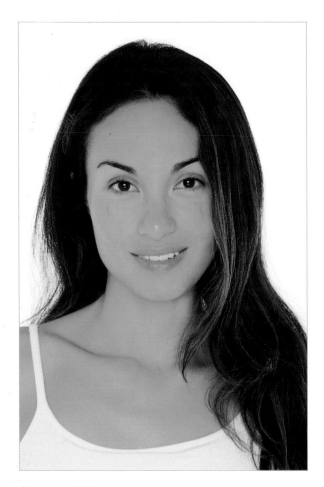

Before and After (facing page)

JULIANA

Juliana is of Hawaiian, Armenian, and Chinese descent, and this unique blend of cultures is responsible for her truly exotic beauty. Her look is so distinctive that she can actually get away with wearing little or no makeup, but she can also go to the opposite extreme and wear quite a lot. Still, she looks best when she wears softer colors to balance out her strong features. Women like Juliana who are lucky enough to be born with really great features don't need to worry so much about using makeup to create optical illusions. My advice if you fall into this category is to use makeup merely as an accessory to make the most of what you have.

I gave Juliana many different looks, but she still looks like Juliana in all of them. I used a lot of different colors, but I took a softer approach. Blending is essential for any natural beauty.

If you'd like to try something dramatic without getting too heavy, pair a deep shade of shadow with a soft, sheer shade of lip color. You can also do a dramatic mouth with a soft, nude eye. No matter what look you choose, avoid hard lines on the eyes and mouth, use soft shades of blush with a little shimmer on top, and blend, blend, blend.

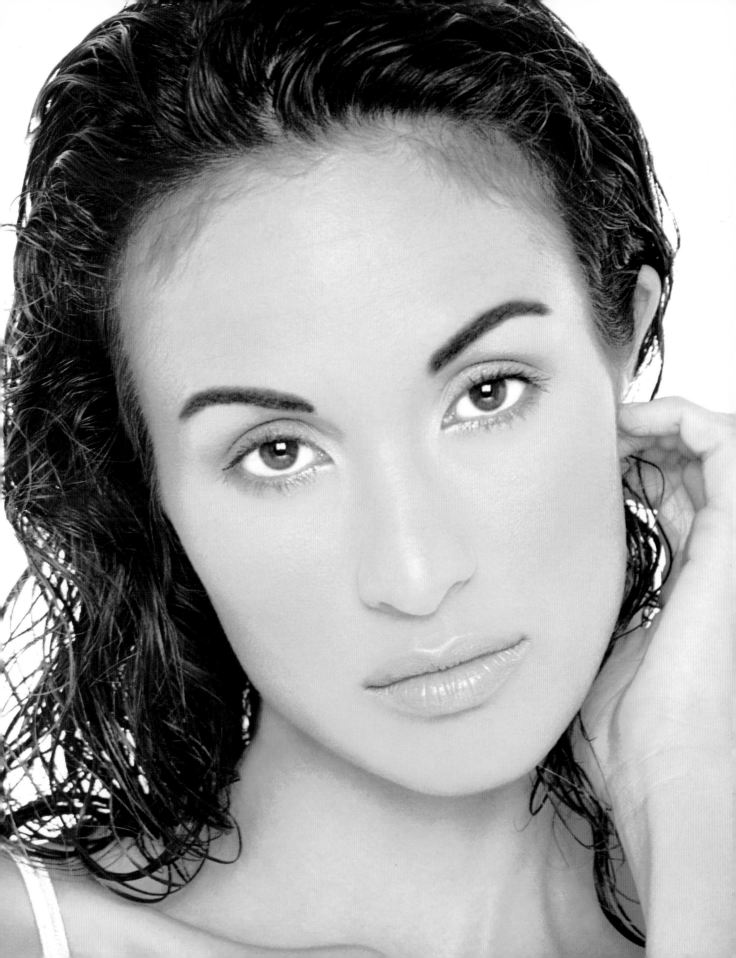

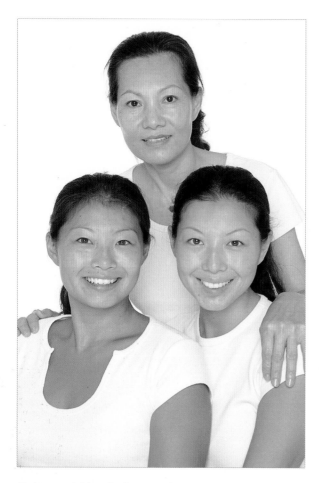

Before and After (facing page)

PRISCILLA, KWOCK LEE, & KYMMI

Imagine my surprise when Priscilla, who is a professional model and actress, showed up for a casting with her younger sister Kymmi in tow. Both of them were absolutely beautiful, and I knew that I wanted to photograph them together. Then they told me about their mother, Kwock Lee, and we decided to do a family portrait. To me these three women are the best examples I could find of timeless beauty. It's obvious that Kwock Lee takes very good care of herself. Her skin is flawless, and her daughters have followed in her footsteps.

Priscilla has three children, and she's very active and outdoorsy. Kymmi, on the other hand, is very feminine. Their mother, who seemed both modest and somewhat shy, nevertheless seemed proud of her age. I didn't think she'd be interested in one of those "Take Ten Years Off" makeovers. To lift her features, I used a little highlighting powder on her cheekbones and at her temples. The whole look was very soft—brown and nutmeg shadow on her eyes and cheeks, oyster highlighter on her brow bone, pale coral lip color.

Priscilla's is a more transparent version of her mother's makeup. Because she's so much younger, she required a lot less foundation. Again, I used soft earth tones on her eyes and lips, just enough color to enhance her natural beauty.

Kymmi's hair is naturally curly, which is quite unusual for an Asian woman. She reminded me of an Asian Veronica Lake, which inspired me to do something a bit more dramatic with her makeup, to emphasize that movie-star quality. Her cheeks are very round, so I contoured them a little, using a darker shade of blush on the lower part of the apples. I also went with a stronger red mouth. She was quite surprised by how she looked when I was done. Before my eyes she seemed to transform from a shy young girl to a sensual young woman, all because of a little paint and powder.

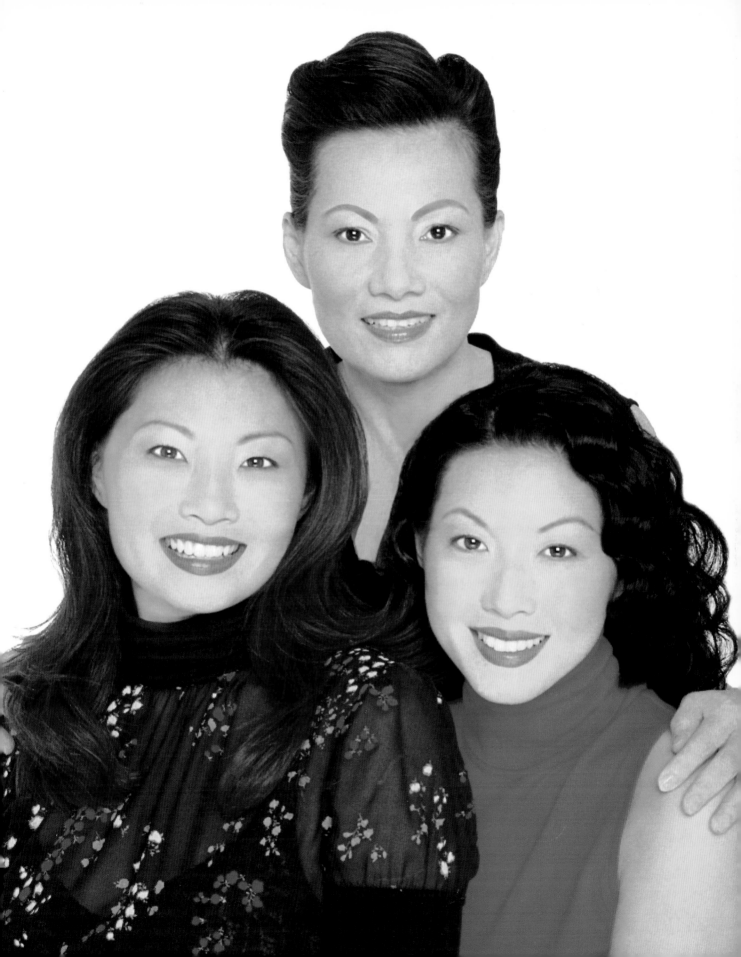

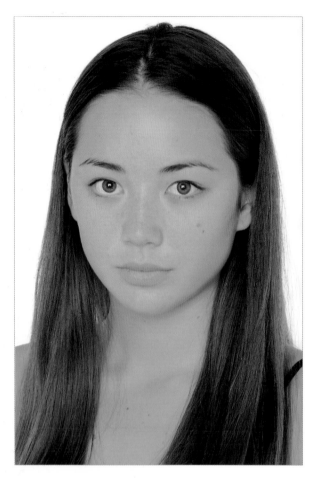

Before and After (facing page)

STEPHANIE

Stephanie, who is sixteen, is young enough to go without makeup and still look good, but she's also at that age when young women really begin to experiment with cosmetics. My best advice is to have fun with makeup but to use transparent colors on the eyes, cheeks, and lids. If your skin is clear, stay away from foundation for as long as possible. If you feel you need a little coverage, try a tinted moisturizer with an SPF. Another option is to apply a little moisturizer, then go over your face with a bit of translucent powder for a flawless finish that doesn't look like a mask. If you have problem skin, a concealer and some dual-finish powder should provide all the coverage you need.

My rule of thumb for young women in general is to keep things sheer. Try cheek gels that blend into the skin rather than formulas that sit on the surface. When choosing eye shadow, try creams instead of powders. They're a lot lighter. If you like a lot of color, use a tinted mascara instead of a lot of heavy color on the eyelid. The important thing is to choose soft colors that work with your skin tone rather than bright, garish shades that make you look much older than you are. This is the one time of your life that you can get away without much makeup. Enjoy it.

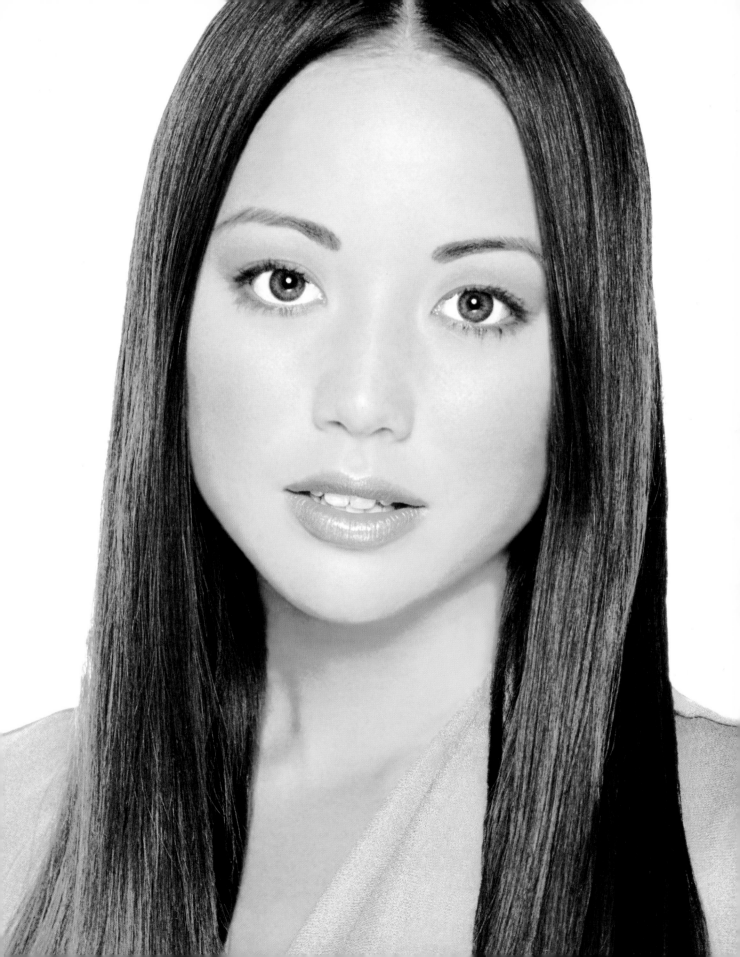

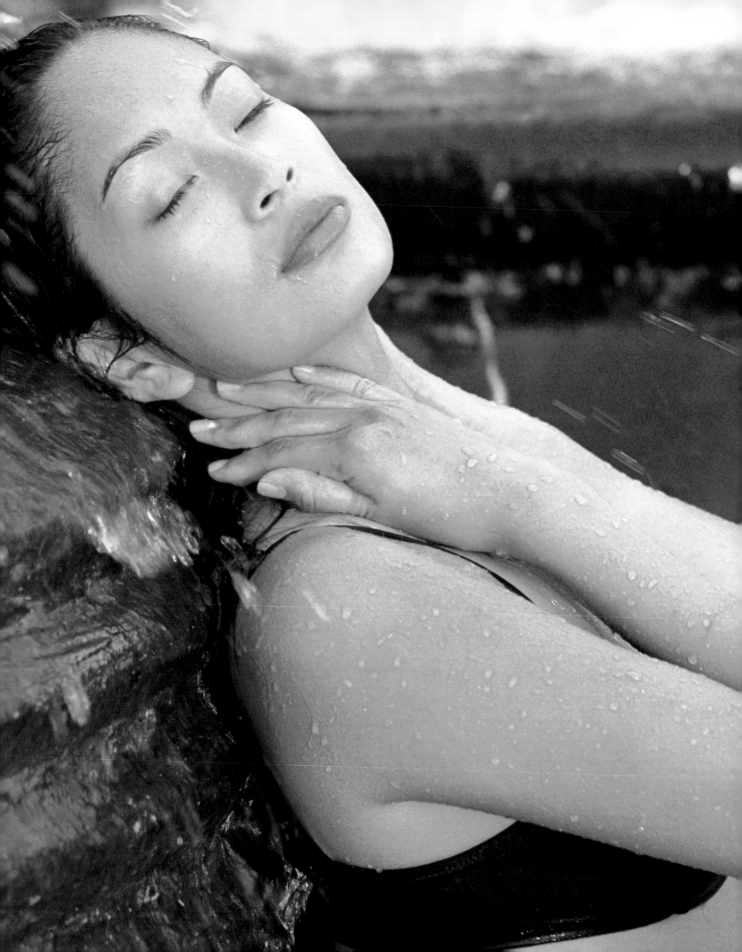

10

BEAUTY INSIDE OUT

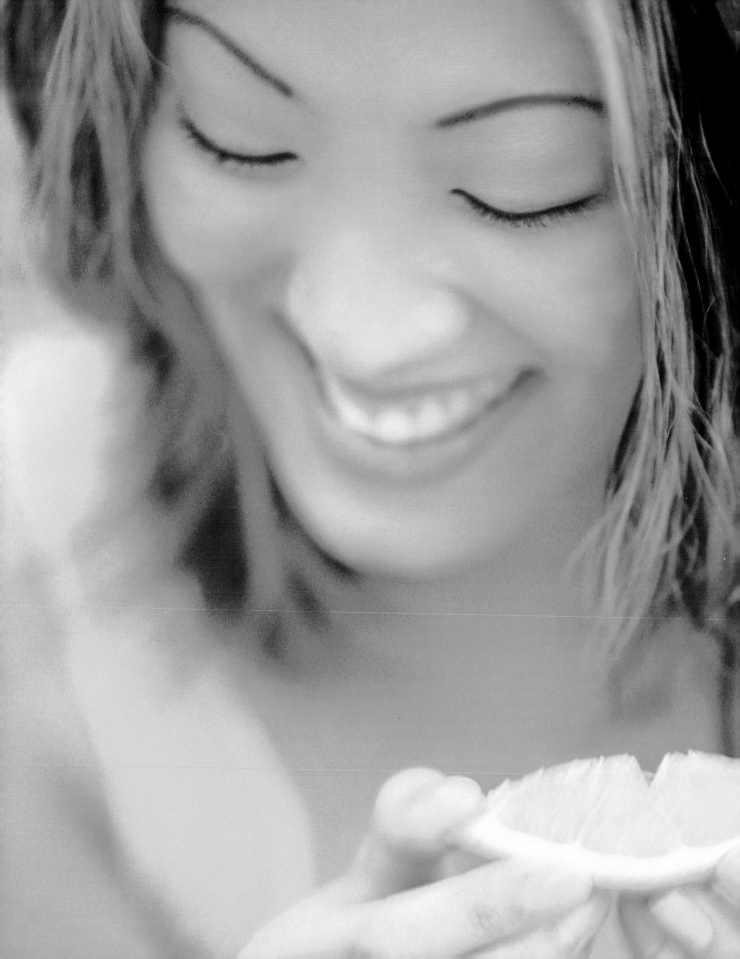

THROUGHOUT MY CAREER I'VE WORKED WITH SOME OF THE MOST BEAUTIFUL PEOPLE IN HOLLYWOOD— WINONA RYDER, GEENA DAVIS, JOAN CHEN, ARNOLD SCHWARZENEGGER, KEVIN COSTNER, MICHAEL JORDAN, AND MEL GIBSON. YOU'VE GOT TO HAVE A PRETTY HEALTHY SELF-IMAGE TO BE SURROUNDED BY ALL THAT PHYSICAL PERFECTION AND NOT FEEL INTIMIDATED. WHAT HELPS IS THAT FOR ME, PHYSICAL BEAUTY IS ONLY HALF OF IT. REAL BEAUTY COMES FROM WITHIN, AND IT HAS A LOT TO DO WITH CONFIDENCE. PEOPLE WHO ARE

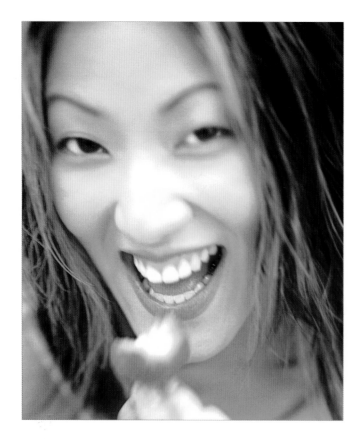

comfortable in their own skins are beautiful to me. Kindness, self-acceptance, strength of character, intelligence—they're all part of what makes a woman beautiful.

It took me years to learn to love myself for who I am. It's all about finding balance in your life, learning to accept the things you cannot change, and changing the things you can. I enjoy sports and fitness—I am an avid hiker and runner—but I have overdone it in the past. I still nurse a knee injury from years of kickboxing. While I realize that working out has become a kind of spiritual outlet for me, I've also learned that I've got to do things in moderation.

Growing up with parents who were born and raised in Japan, I didn't always appreciate how healthy the traditional Japanese diet was, but I like it so much more now. Maybe it's the dairy and the wheat, but my digestive system doesn't do so well on typical American fare.

In her book *Women's Bodies, Women's Wisdom*, Chris Northrup, M.D., one of the few women physicians combining nontraditional healing practices with training as an obstetrician and gynecologist, points out that the United States is one of the few countries in the world where people drink milk well into adulthood. Asian women tend to be lactose-intolerant, which means they've incorporated other sources of calcium into their diet, like soy. Northrup finds a link between diet and breast cancer. Among Japanese women there is a low incidence of breast cancer. But if a Japanese woman were to move to Hawaii, where her diet might consist of a mix of Japanese and American foods, her risk of breast cancer would rise to somewhere between that of Japanese and American women. Even more disturbing is that after she has lived in the United States for eight years, she has the same chance of getting breast cancer as an American woman. Northrup believes that a high-fat Western diet is the culprit.

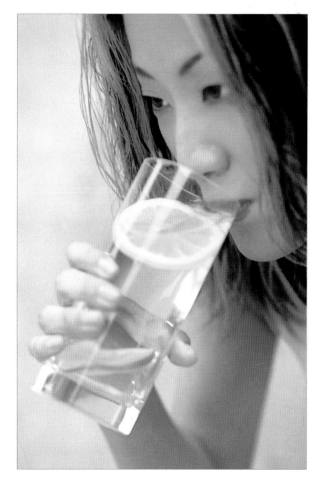

Drinking plenty of water during a rigorous workout is essential for preventing dehydration and replenishing oxygen in the muscles, which increases endurance.

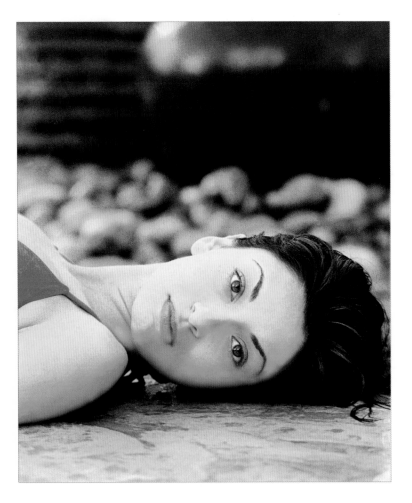

Theresa Gormley, D.C., practices homeopathic medicine at the Los Angeles Center for Healing, which she founded twelve years ago. What she's discovered is that most of us are eating foods that are irritating to our systems. She's concerned that soy, despite its reputation for maintaining hormone levels and keeping bones strong, may have an adverse affect on the thyroid if we're not eating it in combination with vegetables loaded with minerals the thyroid needs in order to thrive. She's not talking about broccoli either. She's talking about sea vegetables, like seaweed and kelp, both of which can be found at the health food store. Her suggestion is to crumble a little dried seaweed on a salad.

Because of our heritage, she says, Asian-American women have a biological need for certain nutrients. It all depends on how Americanized we are and what kind of diet we've eaten most of our lives. The first thing she does is determine what nutrients we're deficient in so she can add those to our diet. Then she deals with any major emotional issues that may be impacting our health. Finally, she performs a chiropractic adjustment to balance the whole system.

I find her approach very much in line with that of my Chinese doctors, who understand the mind/body/spirit connection. In fact, Dr. Gormley is convinced that each of us is on a spiritual journey and that the physical body is a manifestation of what's going on spiritually. By assisting with the nutrition and structure, she believes that she can help the emotional body to be healthy and the soul's vision to be clearer so our journey can continue in a very healthy way.

One of the things I do every morning to strengthen myself both spiritually and emotionally is go walking with my best friend. We both bring our dogs along and spend at least an hour or so hiking in the Hollywood Hills. It's my way of stopping and smelling the roses, so to speak. Anyone who lives in the city understands the importance of finding someplace green to escape to, a place without cell phones, pagers, call waiting, and all of the wonders of modern civilization that make our lives easier but also make them a lot more stressful.

I also find that indulging in simple beauty rituals like taking a bubble bath or having a manicure once a week can do wonders for body and soul. As a makeup artist, I've got to keep my nails short, but I love the way my hands look after I've had a manicure. I'm also a big fan of pedicures, which some people may think are self-indulgent. Actually, there's evidence that taking care of your feet may be good for your health. Keeping your nails

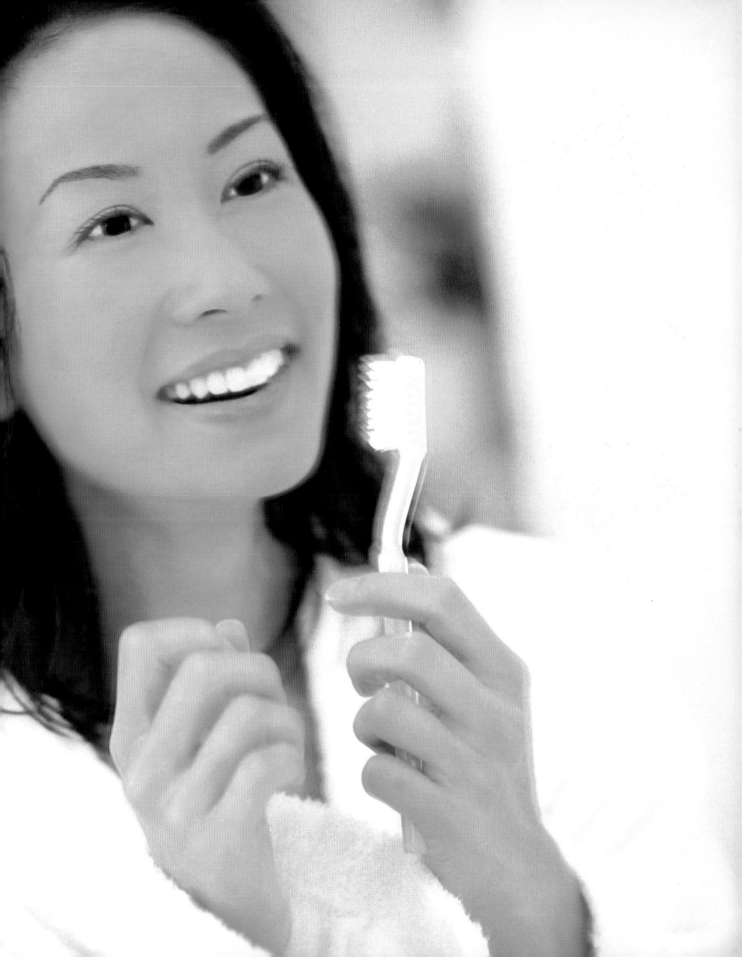

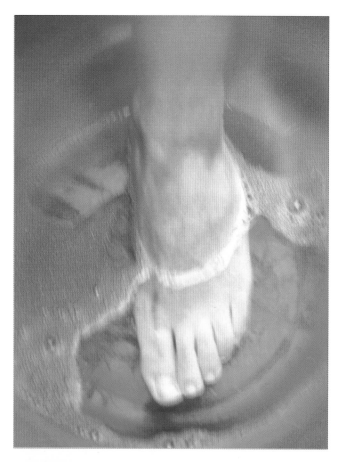

trimmed and buffing calluses may prevent ingrown toenails and improve your posture. Besides, I'm always taking care of everyone else. It's the nature of my job. So it's nice to relax once in a while and let someone else take care of me. I'm sure any woman can relate to that.

I guess what I find important about these little beauty rituals, even the most mundane ones like brushing my teeth or shaving my legs, is that they make me feel good about myself. I'm not suggesting that you become obsessed with how you look, but taking pride in your appearance lets people know that you like who you are.

I didn't always love my body. I was raised to believe that real Asian women don't have breasts or hips, yet I had both. That's why I hated them even when other people complimented me on my curvaceous figure. I tried starvation diets and even managed to whittle myself down to 110 pounds, but I felt terrible. I'm not so sure I looked that great either.

Little beauty rituals, like having a pedicure, shaving my legs, or brushing my teeth make me feel good about myself.

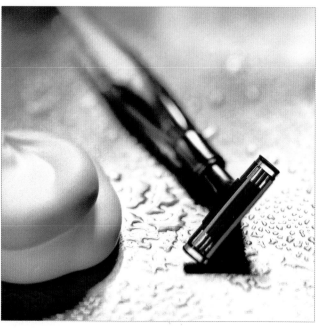

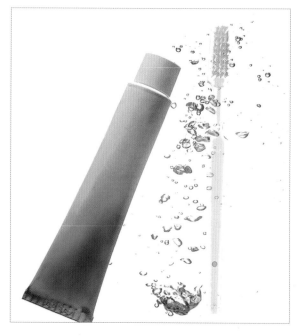

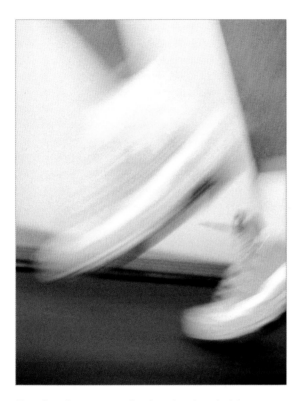

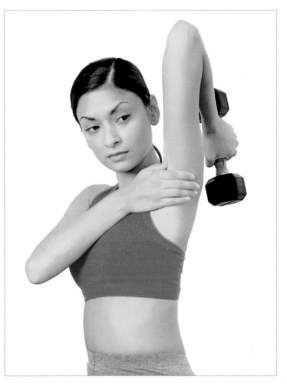

Running keeps me fit, but it also helps me to de-stress.

Working out with weights helps burn fat and works the large muscle groups.

Then about a year and a half ago I met Gary Parker, a personal trainer and exercise physiologist. I had been babying my knee since my injury and was afraid of doing any type of strenuous exercise, but Gary helped me to overcome my fears. He developed a routine for me, a kind of road map that helped me achieve my goals. My big thing was creating obstacles that got in the way, but he challenged me to go further than I ever thought I could. At first I was lucky if I could run a half mile a day, but Gary wouldn't let me coast. He pushed me to run one mile, then two, by telling me stories about the accomplishments of other people who were a lot older than me with more serious injuries.

Now I run between ten and twenty miles per week, depending on my schedule. I always stretch first, which is very important to prevent injuries. I do yoga stretches to open my breathing chakras. It also helps to break down the lactic acid in my muscles, which can cause cramping. Deep breathing helps to relieve stress as well, and Gary is convinced that stress makes me hold on to weight.

Gary also has me working out with weights about three times per week to help burn fat and work the large muscle groups. I do squats for my butt and thighs, arm curls, tricep curls, decline flies to work the chest area, lateral pulldowns for my back and shoulders, and ab work. I usually do three sets of twelve reps with thirty-second breaks between reps.

I always take a bottle of water with me to the gym. Another thing I've learned from Gary is the importance of drinking plenty of water during a rigorous workout. Not only does it prevent dehydration, it helps

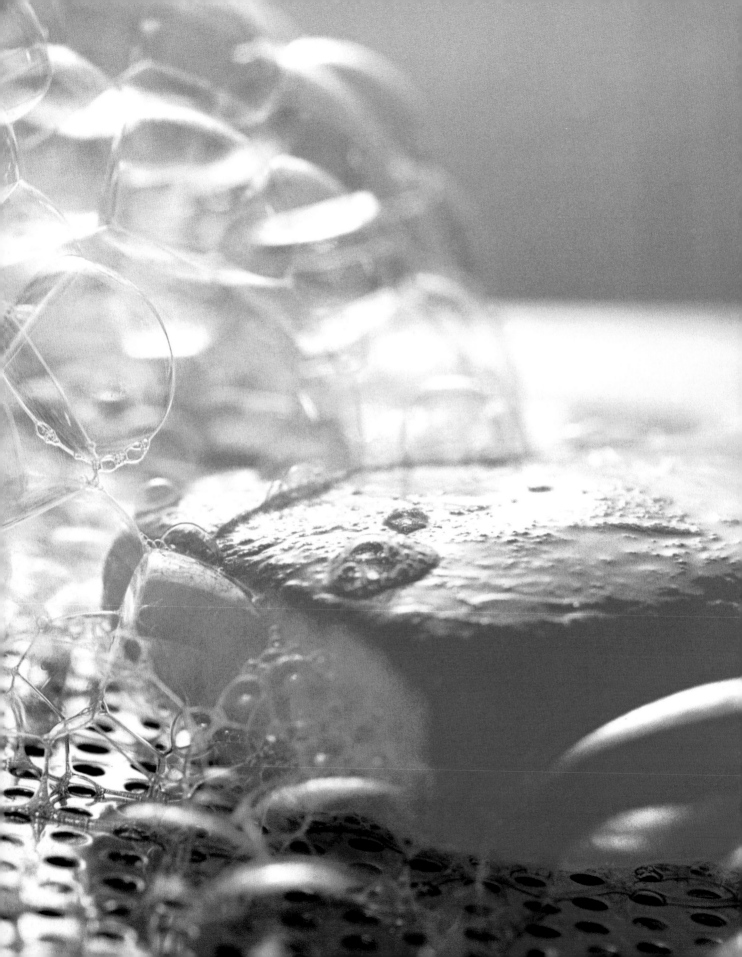

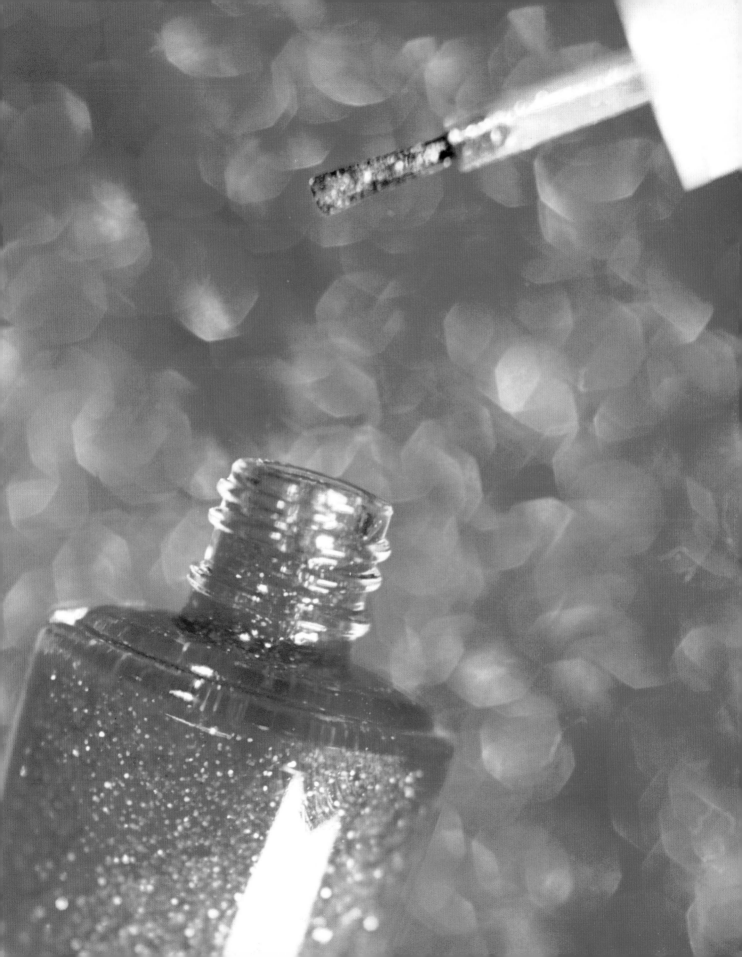

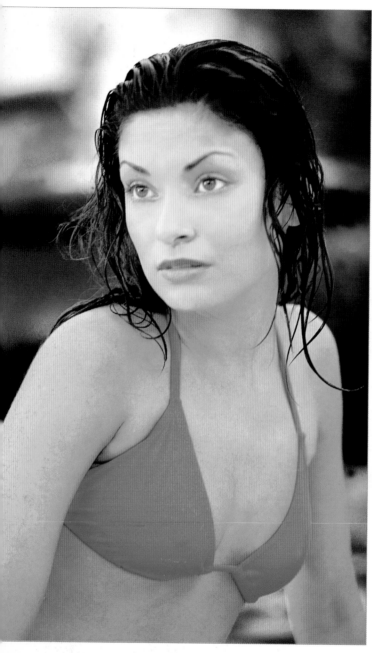

Make the most of what you have instead of focusing on your flaws.

replenish oxygen in the muscles, which increases endurance. If you're one of those people who dislikes the taste of water, invest in bottled spring water and put a slice of lemon in each glass. Post-workout, I have a protein shake or a protein bar to keep my blood sugar level from dipping too low.

At Gary's urging, I also made another lifestyle change. Instead of eating two or three big meals per day, I eat about five smaller meals. I'd been given that advice before, but it never clicked until Gary used this analogy: if you put a big log on the fire in the morning, then throw another big log on six hours later, you'll still have a lot of logs to burn at the end of the day. But if you put a couple of small logs on the fire in the morning, then keep adding other small logs to the fire throughout the day, you'll have nothing left to burn at the end of the day. We can use food in the same way to rev up our metabolism and help us "burn" calories. A lot of small meals throughout the day will use up more energy and burn more calories than a couple of big meals.

It must be working because I'm eighteen pounds lighter and three sizes smaller than I was before. Better yet, I look healthy and fit, and for the first time in my life I love the body I was born with. I'm proud of how strong I am and couldn't care less that I wasn't born with the boyish figure that was the Asian ideal for so long. It's like the way I feel about makeup. You can use it to play up your best features and downplay those you're not so crazy about. If you've got great legs or great shoulders, why not show them off instead of worrying that you'll never have slim hips or a flat chest.

Working out with a friend keeps you motivated.

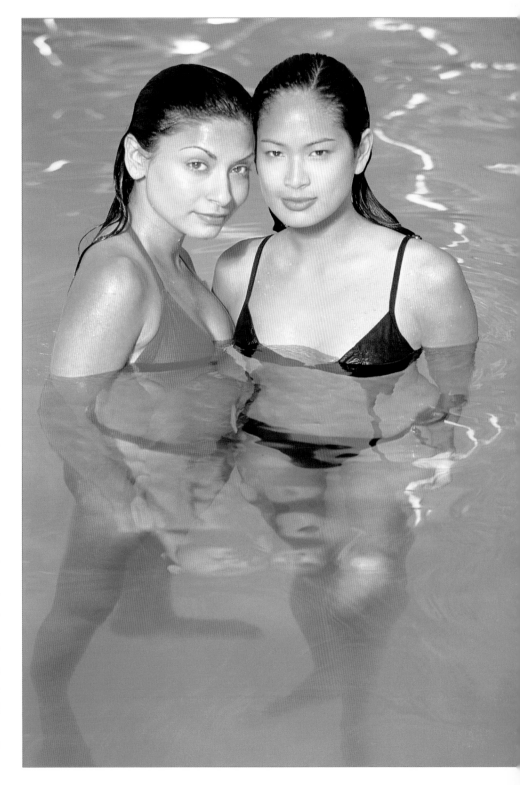

Still, the best thing about becoming fit is that the mental discipline that was required to accomplish my goals has helped me to redefine who I am and what I'm actually capable of. I don't think I could have ever written this book if I hadn't done all this other work on myself first.

When you learn to harness your own power, you'll find that there isn't anything you can't do. I lost my house during the Los Angeles earthquake in 1994. It literally fell down. It's funny though. I loved that house so much that I hadn't noticed how mean most of my neighbors were. But after the earthquake everyone was so nice to each other. The point is, it shouldn't take an earthquake to get you to realize what's important in life.

YOU ARE WHAT YOU EAT

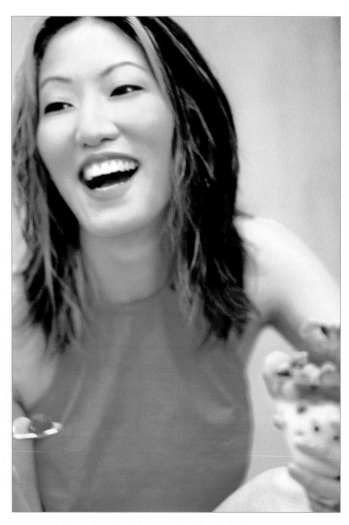

Make the decision to eat fresh fruits and vegetables whenever possible.

I met Leta McCarty twenty years ago when we were both living in Milan. She was a model, and I was a sixteen-year-old makeup artist, but we had a lot in common. Even then Leta was interested in health and nutrition, and we used to come up with these fantastic recipes using tofu, fresh vegetables, and lots of herbs and spices. Eventually Leta went to school to become a holistic nutritionist and organic herbalist. She's still one of my best friends. I rely on her to get me back on track whenever my life gets out of control.

What I like about Leta is that she takes an almost macrobiotic approach to nutrition. The idea is to make seasonal food choices in order to live in harmony with your environment. Let's say it's really cold outside. It's better to eat a bowl of soup or a plate of beans and rice instead of a salad, which just won't prepare you for the harsh environment. But a light spring salad with lots of living enzymes is just what you want to eat on a hot, sunny day. Leta's rule of thumb is to make your main food choices from the food groups that would be available if you lived in the country, not the city with a supermarket just around the corner. The theory is that eating foods that are "in season" will balance your internal thermostat and decrease stress.

One thing I've learned from Leta is to avoid processed foods whenever possible. If you've got a choice, you're always better off with something colorful. Chances are that it has the most living ingredients. And learn to read labels. Red flags include fat, sugar, and textured vegetable protein. Artificial and chemical additives are just as bad. Our bodies just aren't set up to process them and will actually store them in our fatty tissue, where they become cellulite.

We all have excuses that keep us from making healthy choices, but making the effort to eat right will pay off in the long run. Your skin will look more radiant, you'll have more energy, and you'll probably live longer too. Here are some suggestions to help you rethink the way you eat:

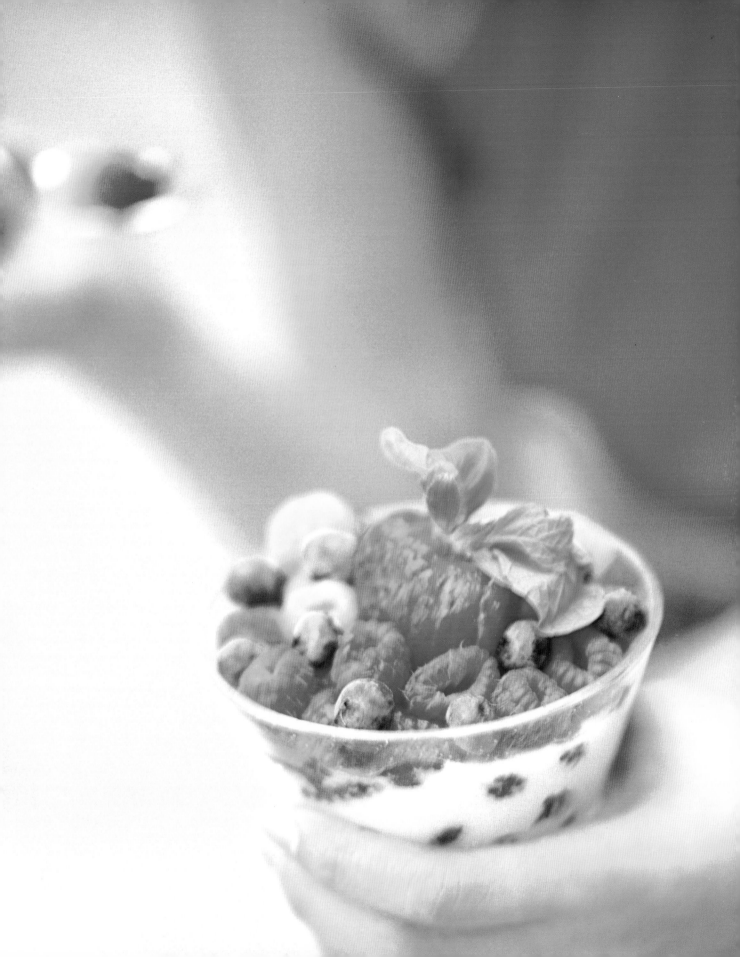

* On a budget? Make a pot of beans and rice that can take you through the week.

* Base your diet on three multicolored vegetables per meal plus a lean protein (fish, soy, or small beans or legumes).

* If you're a vegetarian, add beans to golden and green vegetables to create a balanced protein.

* Use Sunday as meal preparation day. That way you'll have something in the fridge when you get home from work so you'll be less likely to order a pizza instead.

* Marinate poultry, fish, or tofu and store in freezer bags. Leave one in the refrigerator to thaw while you're at work, then stick it under the broiler at night.

* Check health food stores, whole food stores, or the freezer section of your grocery store for edamame (Japanese soy beans). They're the highest quality of soy protein available.

* Avoid veggie burgers that are full of textured protein, fat, or artificial or chemical additives. Boca Burgers, which are high in protein and low in fat, are a much better choice.

* Make a salad of multicolored vegetables that will last three or four days (radish, leaf lettuce, purple cabbage, carrots, sugar snap peas). Store in plastic containers in the refrigerator. Add bell pepper, tomato, or cucumber the day you use it.

* Make a pot of soup using six multicolored vegetables—white onions, green beans, purple potatoes, yellow squash, bright orange carrots, and juicy red tomatoes. Add water, spices, herbs, and a protein source like beans, tofu, fish, or chicken. For best results, add spices like garlic, cumin, or chili powder at the beginning of the preparation and fresh or dried herbs like basil or rosemary at the end.

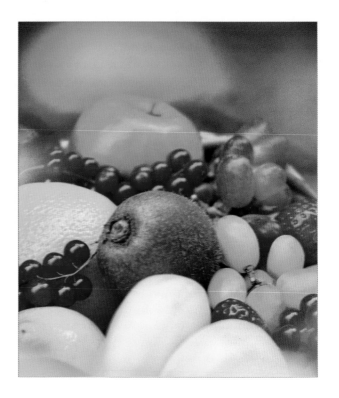

I know this is easier said than done, but once you muster the willpower to make conscious choices, you'll actually recondition your craving for the kind of food that provides the most immediate gratification and will feel satisfied.

THE BREAKFAST CLUB

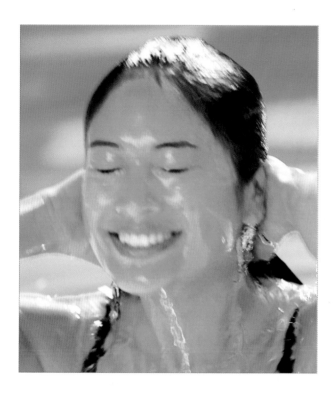

One way to increase your energy, control your cravings, and balance your elimination is to satisfy your cellular nutritional needs the first thing in the morning. Leta taught me to start my day with a green drink or protein shake. Here are the recipes:

GREEN DRINK: You can get a green powder (powdered algae and sea vegetables) at any health food store. It's high in antioxidants, micro and macro minerals, and B vitamins, plus the chlorophyll acts as a natural filter for the digestive system and blood. My favorite is a product called Greens Plus—it doesn't clump. Mix a spoonful with organic apple juice or add a tablespoon to your protein shake.

PROTEIN SHAKE: Place the following ingredients in a blender, and blend until smooth:

1 serving of soy- or whey-based PROTEIN POWDER

1 tbsp. GREENS PLUS

1 tbsp. FLAXSEED OIL (essential fatty acids)

½ tsp. PROBIOTIC ACIDOPHILUS or ¼ cup plain UNSWEETENED YOGURT

½ cup fresh or frozen BERRIES

1 BANANA

10 oz. organic APPLE JUICE or SOY MILK

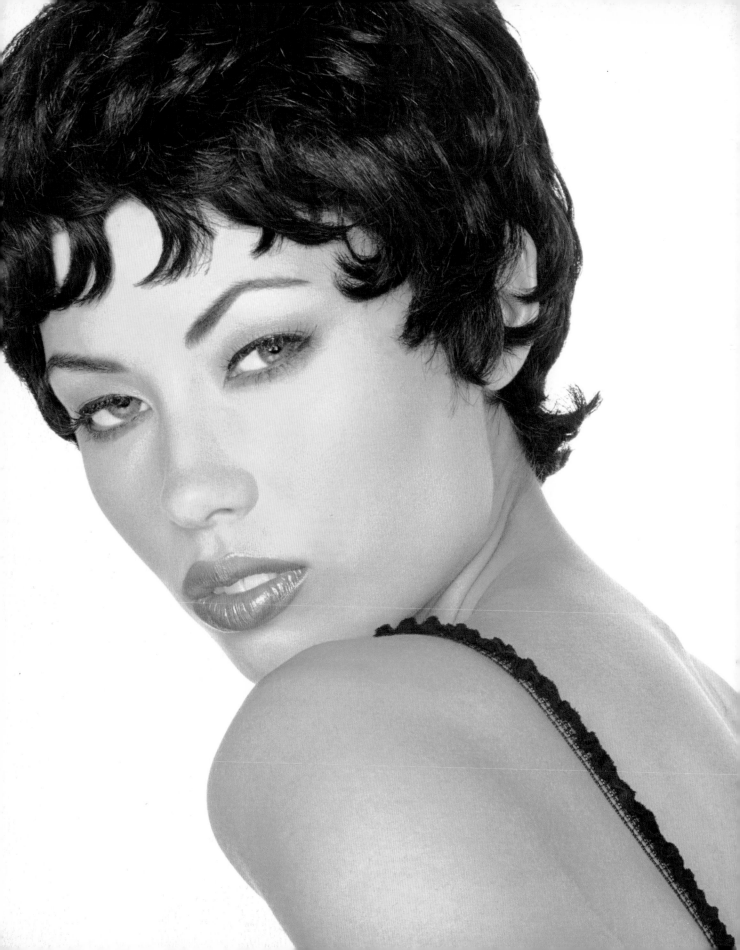

GET A NEW ATTITUDE

11

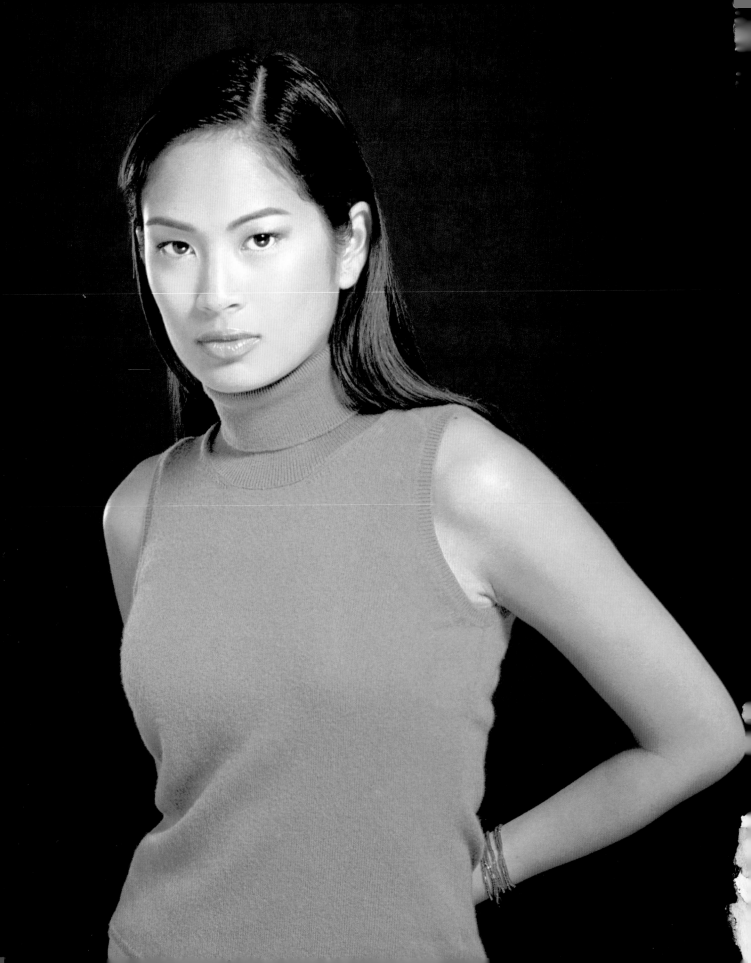

IN MY TWENTY YEARS AS A PROFESSIONAL MAKEUP ARTIST, I HAVE DEVELOPED A SIXTH SENSE FOR READING PEOPLE, AND I CAN TELL A LOT ABOUT SOMEONE BY THEIR APPEARANCE. THIS MAY SOUND SUPERFICIAL, BUT IT'S NOT. EVERYTHING FROM THE WAY YOU WEAR YOUR HAIR TO WHETHER YOU POLISH YOUR SHOES SPEAKS VOLUMES ABOUT YOUR SENSE OF SELF-WORTH. IT MAY BE A CLICHÉ, BUT IT'S WORTH REPEATING: YOU DON'T GET A SECOND CHANCE TO MAKE A FIRST IMPRESSION. BUT EVEN IF

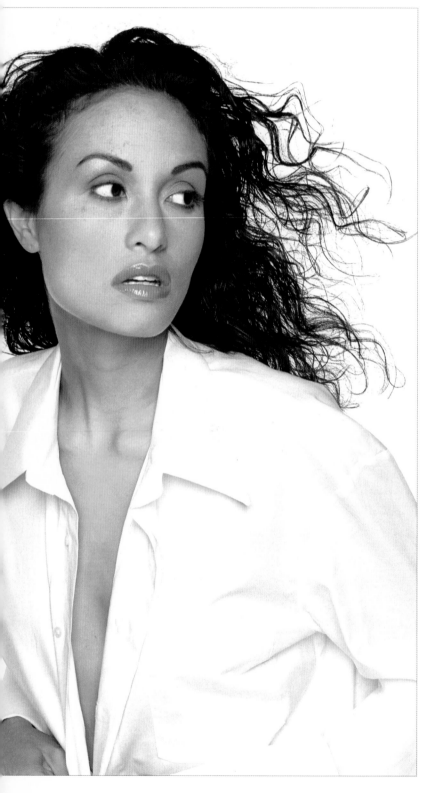

you've got $300 highlights in your hair, the latest Prada handbag on your arm, and Jimmy Choo stilettos on your feet, you're not going to impress anyone if you don't like who you are. It's another cliché but one that also applies here: beauty is only skin-deep. I believe that. Real beauty comes from within. Attitude is everything. Do you really like who you are? Do you even know who you are? If not, it's time to start developing some skills that can help you live a happier, more fulfilled life. That way, when you're ready for your close-up, people will really like what they see.

✳ **MAKE TIME FOR YOURSELF:** Set aside an hour and a half a day for yourself. Do something that makes you happy, whether it's soaking in a warm bath, taking a yoga class, or having dinner with a friend. And set aside one full day a week for R&R. Even God rested on the seventh day. More important, do not break these rules for anyone. If you don't take care of yourself, you won't be much good to anyone else.

✳ **SET GOALS:** Start simple to build your confidence, then gradually set loftier goals. Let's say you want to eliminate sweets from your diet. Instead of swearing off sweets for good, try to get through one day without them. When you accomplish this relatively simple goal, try to get through a week, then a month. There's less chance of failure when you set realistic goals for yourself and discover that you can actually accomplish something you set out to do.

✳ **START A JOURNAL:** This is a great way to make friends with yourself. Most of us fill our days with endless activities that keep us from

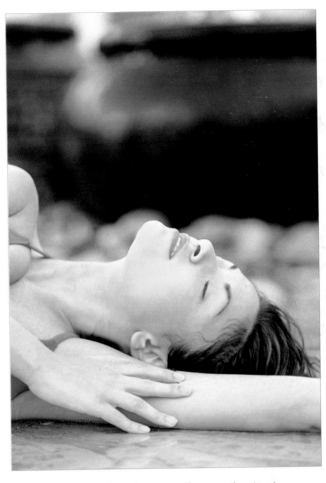

Set aside some time for yourself every day to do something that makes you happy.

spending any time alone. Use your journal to vent your frustrations or to explore your deepest fears, to record events that happen and examine how they made you feel. As time goes by, you will start to see improvements in all areas of your life. When Socrates said, "The unexamined life is not worth living," he knew what he was talking about. It's important to write something every day, even if it's just a word or two. Make journaling a habit, like brushing your teeth and washing your face before you go to bed at night. Think of it as weight lifting for the soul. The only way you'll see results is if you do it religiously.

✳ **LEARN TO FORGIVE:** Holding a grudge inevitably hurts you more than it hurts the person you're angry with. Anger just makes us mean or keeps us down. If you blame your parents or your husband or your sister for something they've done to hurt you, find it in your heart to forgive them. Then let it go. This might sound simplistic, even unrealistic, but it works. Sometimes we blame ourselves for things we've done, like cheating on our diet or losing our temper, and we punish ourselves for it. But blame is a negative emotion, and besides, no one's perfect. Once you accept that fact, you'll find it a lot easier to forgive. That alone can help you have a more positive outlook.

✳ TAKE RESPONSIBILITY: Unfortunately it's human nature to pass the buck. You'll be happier in the long run if you learn to take responsibility for your actions. The idea is to make conscious decisions about everything you do and only do those things that you have reverence for.

✳ DARE TO DO SOMETHING DIFFERENT: We all have dreams and aspirations, but how many of us actually do something to make those dreams come

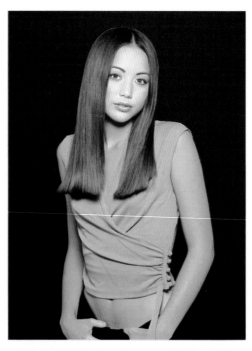

Use a journal to vent your frustrations or explore your deepest fears.

true? Some of us spend so much time trying to live up to someone else's expectations that we forget what it was that we wanted to be when we grew up. Or we get bogged down in the routine of daily life. We don't believe it's possible to change our circumstances, to move to the country or live near the ocean or take piano lessons at forty or learn how to become a pastry chef after years of being a first-grade teacher. My advice is to decide what you really, really want, then go for it. It's important to be realistic. After all, you're probably never going to be a prima ballerina if you have two left feet. Well, you know what I mean. But if you believe in your heart that you can do something, then you probably can. It's worth finding out, isn't it?

✳ LEARN TO LOVE YOURSELF NAKED: This might seem impossible and it will almost certainly take time, but it will transform your life in ways you never imagined.

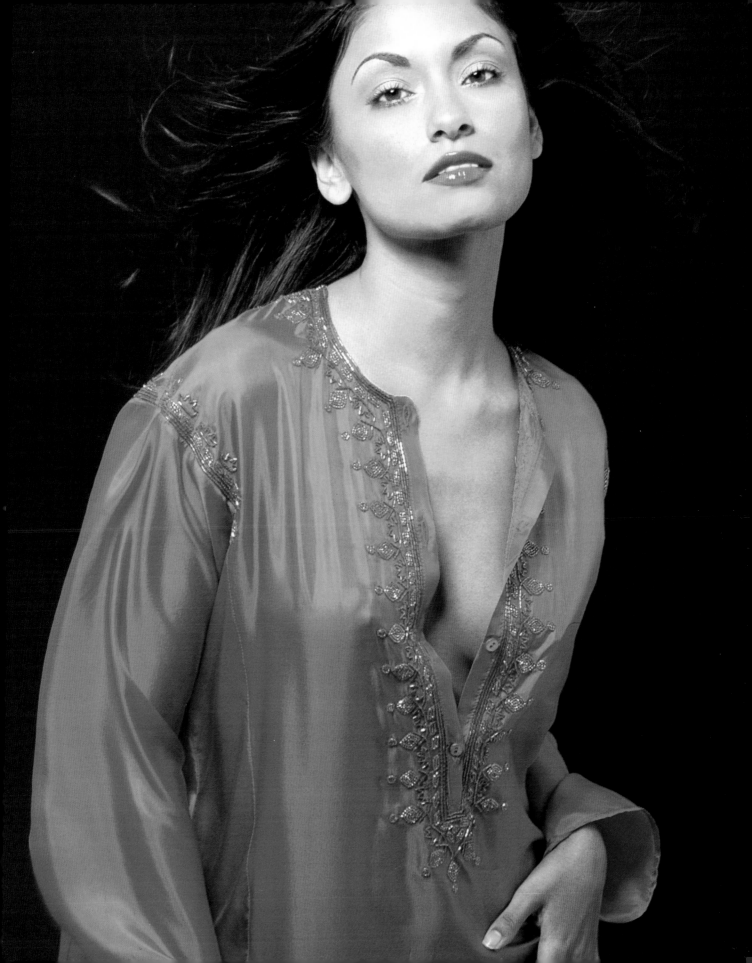

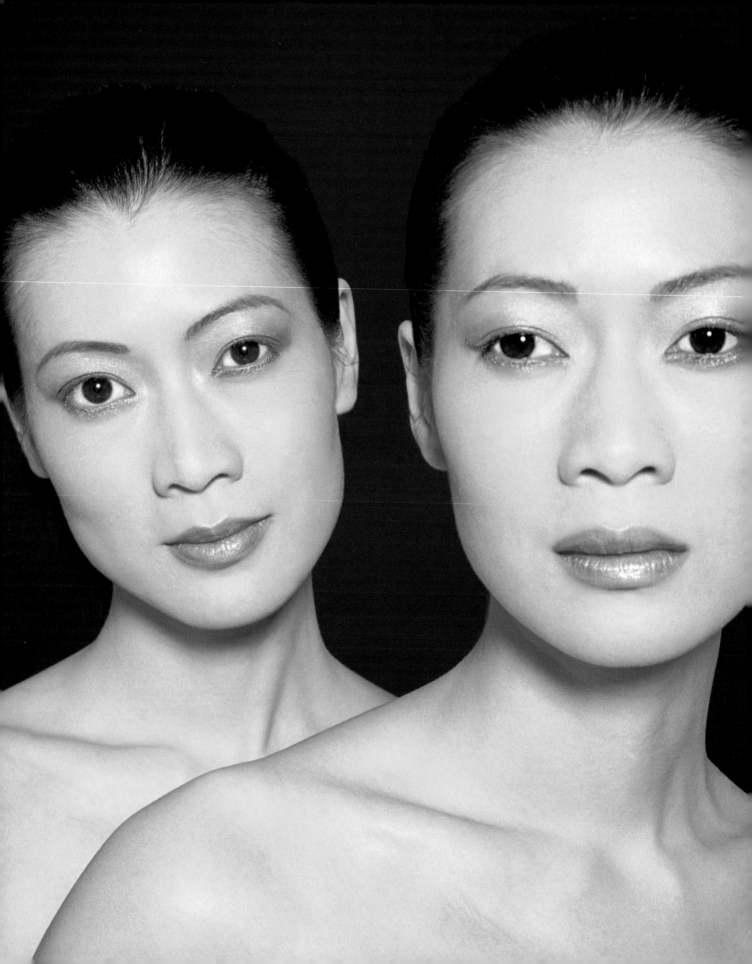

A C K N O W L E D G M E N T S

Thank you, God, for the gifts of trust, hope, love, and faith. You have taught me "If you don't go within, you go without."

Words cannot express my appreciation to my family for all of their unconditional love and support.

Kyoko, Yumi, Mari, Bill, and Wendy, thank you.

Thank you to my father, who encouraged us never to get a 9-to-5 job.

I would like to thank the following people for their continual love and support:

Gary Parker for teaching me to believe in faith. This world would be flat without you. Thanks, Sweetie.

Rich Marchewka for all of your infinite talents. You will always be my little brother.

Larisa Jenkins for being my canyon spiritual soul sister. You have been a great teacher.

Gert for your encouragement and loving friendship.

Ann Lewis for your heart of gold. You are one of the most talented people I will ever know.

Yu Hayami (Kami) for always being there when I needed you.

I would also like to thank Julie, Kristen and Bill, Alice, Tammy-Indie, Janine, Gregory, Kia, Shirley, Bill Imada, Ken, Denise, Leta McCarty, Margo Peck, Katie Williams, Richard T. Higashi, Errol Navickas, Alan Bair, Joseph Lomeli, Aimee Candelaria, Dylan Gordon, Terrance and Conny, and especially Andie (Rose) McDowell for providing me with a make-up kit, just when I was about to walk away from the whole thing. There are many of you I did not mention, but you know who you are.

Thanks to my partners, Meiko Ajiro and Andrew Yap, and my staff for their loving support, with a special thanks to Sherri Azad for her hard work and dedication, and to Paula Jane Hamilton for her constant assistance.

Very deep-felt thanks to Jeni Chua, Shelly Kamanitz, Sandra Savanpredi, and Kim Sakamoto for being there and believing in my dream.

Thank you, Jessica Wainwright, for your faith in me. Your conviction is immeasurable.

Thank you, Marianne Dougherty, for your insight and craftsmanship. I will forever cherish our spiritual conversations.

I'd like to thank everyone at HarperCollins for all of their hard work. A heartfelt thank-you to my editor, Ayesha Pande, for all of her patience and support in making sure this book reflected my true intentions.

Thank you, Nick Darrell, for being there when I needed someone to help me. Your hard work will never be taken for granted.

I'd also like to thank Susan Kosko, Karen Lumley, Leah Carlson-Stanisic, and Megan Newman, as well as the entire PR and marketing departments.

Thank you to everyone at Bragman Nyman and Caferelli, especially to Sarah Young, who has been such a dear support system, and to Jeri-Anne for her great assistance. Thank you Nadine Ono for your hard work and dedication. Thanks to the Cloutier Agency for their constant support and encouragement. It has been a great, long journey.

Thank you, Arnold Schwarzenegger, for teaching me that there is a creative process to business.

Thank you, Lisa Ling, for your beauty, brains and support. Your participation in this project means so much to me.

Thank you, Mary and Laura Ling.

Thanks to all of the beautiful women who are in this book, especially to Ria and Therese Rueda, Jeannie Hart, Joomi Ha, Sharon Tay, and Jordan Goldstein.

A very special thanks to Cheryl Tan and Shazia Ali for the extra mile you've gone for me.

Thank you to Champaign Trott, Nous, and Elite.

A special thanks to Mark and Emily Goldstein and "EmmaGold" for all of the beautiful clothes, and to Lisa and Frank Glasso at Frank Studios for the studio space, and to "T" and Nam for their talents, which helped accomplish my dream.

Thank you to Steve Block and A&I color lab. I truly appreciate you for believing in this project.

I'd like to thank Peter Alvarez for his beautiful hair magic and endless jokes, as well as Toby Tilley for his beautiful still-life images.

I'd also like to thank Mark Belgraph at Belle de Jour for the beautiful products and locations, as well as for your kindness and endless support.

Thank you to the Paint Shop Nail Spa for the manicures.

Thank you Robertson Optical and Akbar and Roshi.

Thank you to the premier of Sherman Oaks.

Thank you, Los Angeles Center for Healing, Anna Marie Colavito, Felicia Perez, Tina Lynne, and Dr. Theresa Gormley, for all of your help and amazing insight.

Thank you, Helen Famularé, spa-training manager at the Elizabeth Arden Red Door Salon and Spa in Manhattan, for your sound advice.

Thank you, Charles Spilo of Spilo Worldwide, Los Angeles, for the Rubis tweezers.

Last, I would like to thank all of my great teachers who have supplied me with sensibility and discernment.

Thank you, Oprah Winfrey, for being my muse.

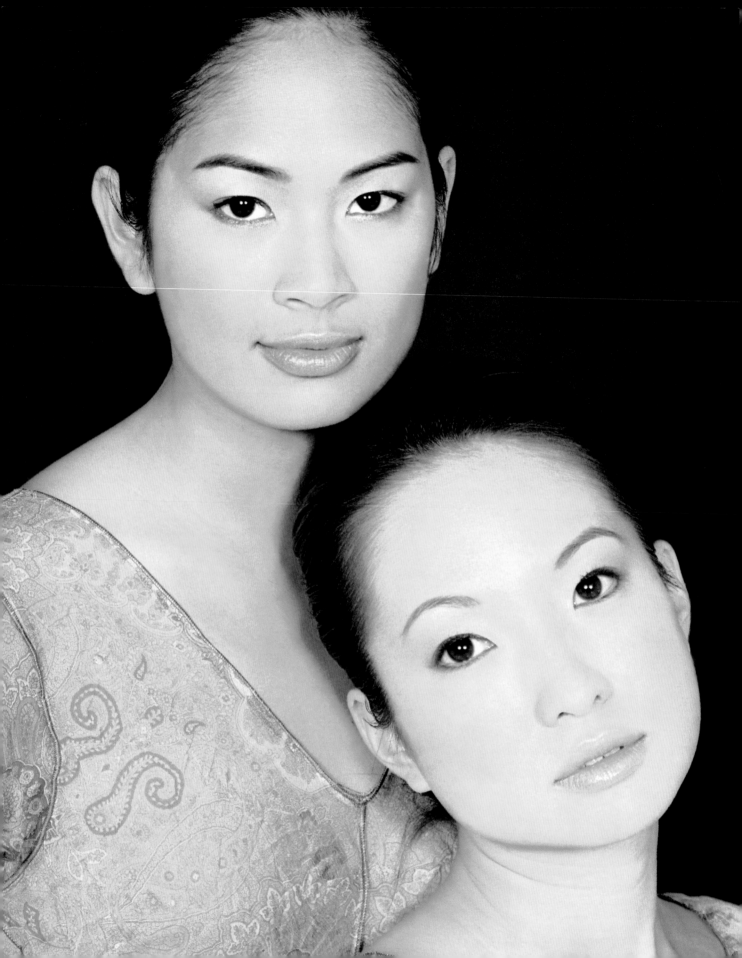

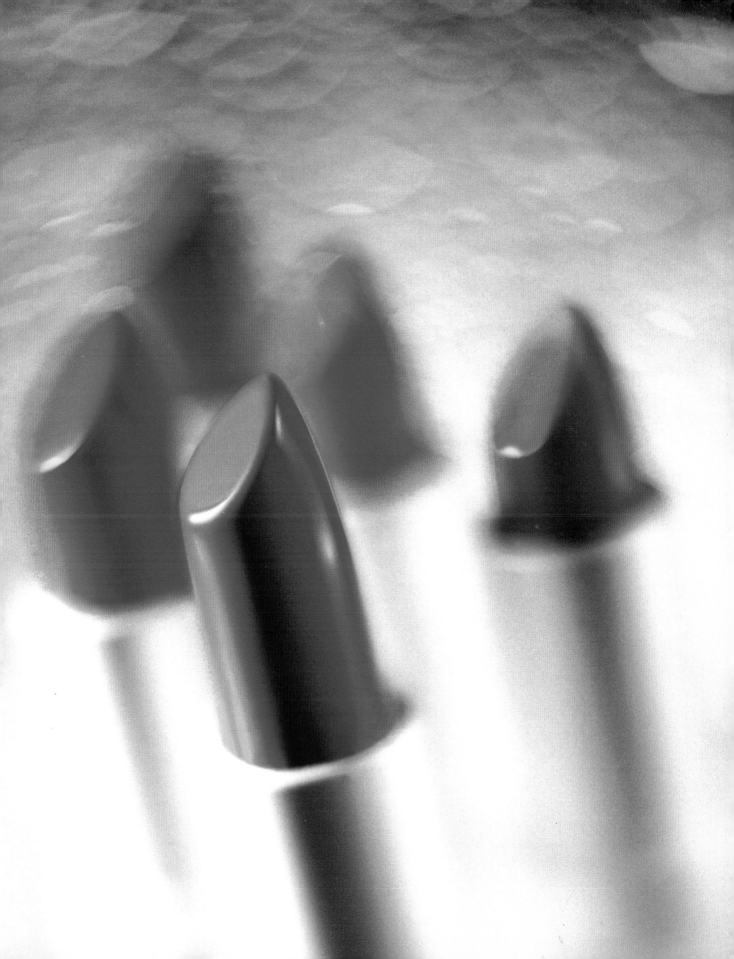

ABOUT THE AUTHORS

MARGARET KIMURA is a veteran image-maker and a professional makeup artist who has been working in the fashion and entertainment industries for the past twenty years. During her career she has worked with such celebrities as Audrey Hepburn, Arnold Schwarzenegger, Tom Hanks, and Andie MacDowell.

Margaret has worked in Milan, Paris, Tokyo, New York, and Hollywood. Throughout she found that, as an Asian-American woman, it was difficult to find cosmetics and application methods appropriate for Asian women. Therefore she decided to develop her own line of cosmetics, Margaret Kimura Cosmetics. Margaret is a native Californian who lives in Los Angeles.

MARIANNE DOUGHERTY is an award-winning writer and beauty editor. She is the former publisher of *American Salon* and *American Spa* magazines and the former editor in chief of *Shades of Beauty*. She has appeared as a beauty consultant on *Live in L.A.*, the Lifetime Network's *New Attitudes*, and *Weekend Today in New York*. She lives in Pittsburgh, where she is at work on a novel.

RICH MARCHEWKA is an award-winning travel photographer and photojournalist whose work has taken him all over the world. He has worked with the White House and USAID to create images to raise awareness of the devastating AIDS epidemic in Africa and the still-growing epidemic in the United States. The International Library of Photography has published his work, and his images have also appeared in magazines such as *W*, *Honey*, *Shades of Beauty*, *Metropolis*, *American Photo*, and *Islands Magazine*. Recent work includes advertising images for Margaret Kimura Cosmetics. He lives in Los Angeles.